THE HEAD-INJURED COLLEGE STUDENT

THE HEAD-INJURED COLLEGE STUDENT

By

COOPER B. HOLMES, PH.D.

Professor of Psychology
Emporia State University
Private Practice of Neuropsychology
Emporia, Kansas

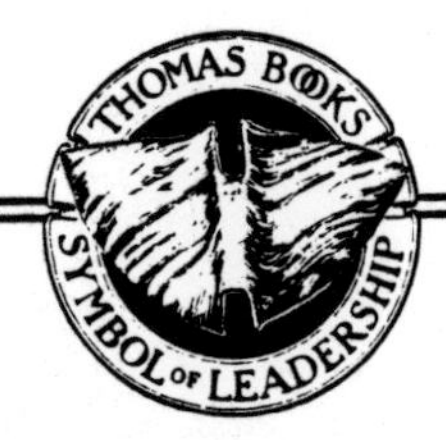

CHARLES C THOMAS • PUBLISHER
Springfield • Illinois • U.S.A.

Published and Distributed Throughout the World by

CHARLES C THOMAS • PUBLISHER
2600 South First Street
Springfield, Illinois 62794-9265

ISBN 0-398-05475-4

Library of Congress Catalog Card Number: 88-2277

With THOMAS BOOKS *careful attention is given to all details of manufacturing and design. It is the Publisher's desire to present books that are satisfactory as to their physical qualities and artistic possibilities and appropriate for their particular use.* THOMAS BOOKS *will be true to those laws of quality that assure a good name and good will.*

Printed in the United States of America
Q-R-3

Library of Congress Cataloging in Publication Data

Holmes, Cooper B.
The head-injured college student.

Bibliography: p.
Includes index.
1. Brain damage. 2. College students—Wounds and injuries. 3. College students—Mental health services. I. Title. [DNLM: 1. Brain Injuries. 2. Student Health Services—United States. WL 354 H749h]
RC387.5.H65 1988 617'.481044 88-2277
ISBN 0-398-05475-4

This book is dedicated to Charles Dee Packer (1920-1980), Judith Raye Wiley Holmes (1942-1982) and Velma Clarice Hartzler (1921-1987).

ACKNOWLEDGMENTS

I WOULD LIKE to acknowledge Michael E. Howard, Ph.D., a former student who became my teacher in neuropsychology. Without the excellent training I received from Dr. Howard I would not have attempted this book. I must thank Dee Ann Holmes for helping make the postdoctoral training possible.

I would also like to acknowledge the participants at the September, 1987 meeting of the Kansas Head Injury Association. Their interest and questions helped show the need for a book on the head-injured college student.

C.B.H.

CONTENTS

THE HEAD-INJURED COLLEGE STUDENT

CHAPTER 1

INTRODUCTION

DEFINITION OF HEAD INJURY

MANY TERMS are used to describe the variety of ways the human brain may become impaired. There are congenital problems, those present at birth, and acquired brain injury (ABI). Traumatic brain injury (TBI) is an injury acquired as a result of some trauma such as an accident. Terms such as brain dysfunction and brain impairment are used, but both refer to the same thing. One is likely to be perplexed by such terms as brain insult and brain lesion, both of which refer to *any* type of brain injury from accidents to tumors to strokes.

To maintain consistency throughout this book the term head injury will be used to describe all forms of brain impairments, regardless of cause or severity. Using the term head injury in this way is the best single way to encompass all disorders.

SCOPE OF THE PROBLEM

Obtaining accurate information on the number of head-injured individuals is difficult. Figures are reported that range from 400,000 to 700,000 new cases per year which result in hospitalization (National Head Injury Foundation, 1985; Begali, 1987). Rosenthal (1987) placed the number of hospitalized head injuries at 500,000. He noted that between 30,000 and 50,000 of these cases are physically or neurobehaviorally unable to return to their pre-injury level of functioning. Unfortunately for the person seeking complete information, the previously noted figures refer only to hospitalized cases. We have no definitive data on the number of head injury cases that are not hospitalized. Caveness

(1979) estimated there are about 7,000,000 cases of head injury per year. Matthews (1987) estimated a yearly rate of 6,000,000 head injuries in children under 16 years of age, and that 1,000,000 of these are major injuries. According to data from the United States Department of Health and Human Services (1984) males are twice as likely to incur a head injury, and the most frequent age range for head injuries is between 15 and 24 years, accounting for approximately two-thirds of all head injury cases. Not surprisingly, automobile accidents are the major cause of head injuries in this age group.

The enormity of the problem becomes apparent when we consider that the data reflect only the reported cases. Available information allows no inference about how many people suffer head injuries that go unreported and untreated. Recent research has shown an alarming result: even minor head injuries, those with less than 20 minutes unconsciousness and brief or no hospitalization, produce significant aftereffects. Rimel, Giordini, Barth, Boll, and Jane (1981) studied over 500 cases of minor head injury and found impairments such as confusion and memory loss lasting up to three months post-injury, with a subsequent unemployment rate of 34 percent. Mersky and Woodforde (1972) studied 27 psychiatric patients with minor head injuries and found mental symptoms lasting a median of four years post-injury. Consider these data in light of Marshall and Marshall's (1985) estimate that 300,000 people are hospitalized each year for minor head injuries.

It is staggering to imagine the potential number of people who have incurred a minor head injury (or a series of such injuries) who never sought medical attention. It is equally staggering to imagine the number of people who did get medical attention after a minor head injury but who were not told of potential aftereffects because, at the time, the aftereffects were not known. As our level of knowledge increases, we are becoming more and more aware of how little it takes to cause brain damage. Recalling the largest number of head injuries occur in the 15 to 24 year age range, and the very likely large number of unreported cases, it is apparent that the educational system must address the needs of head-injured students.

THE RESPONSE OF PUBLIC EDUCATION

Begali (1987) estimated the rate of head-injured public school children in the United States to be roughly 150 to 550 per 100,000 population.

The educational system in the United States has been slow in responding to the needs of head-injured students, but recent trends are encouraging (National Head Injury Foundation, 1985). In general, the fields of behavioral neurology, neuropsychology (psychologists specifically trained to work with head-injured persons), and head-injury rehabilitation are growing rapidly, and along with them the material on head-injured students. There are many excellent articles and books on this topic (Begali, 1987; Golden & Anderson, 1979; Hartlage & Telzrow, 1985; National Head Injury Foundation, 1985; Ylivsaker, 1985). In addition, there are excellent information sources such as the National Head Injury Foundation and local and state head injury associations. Their information presents clear explanations of the nature of head injury and how to plan an educational program around the injury. It is premature to say that the educational system has all the available resources it needs, but there is certainly a growing body of literature on the topic.

RESOURCES ON THE HEAD-INJURED COLLEGE STUDENT

The prevalence of material on the head-injured public school student (pre-school to high school) unfortunately does not extend to the head-injured college student. College here refers to two-year junior or community colleges or to four-year colleges and graduate schools. Through various sources, resource centers, meetings and personal contacts I know there are many college personnel specifically working with head-injured students. Unfortunately, much of their work is largely unknown to the educational system as a whole, and almost nothing is written in the form of articles and books. Some seminars and presentations have been tape recorded and are available (Savage, Cohen, Coyne, Fryer, & Harrington, 1985; Cook, Knight, & Harrington, 1986; Cook & Knight, 1987; Holmes, 1987), but even these are not widely known to the majority of people working with head-injured persons who are students or who are potential college students.

The material in neuropsychology, neurology, education, and rehabilitation provides anecdotal material (reports, case studies, personal accounts) rather than research results. This lack of research extends to even the most basic facts about the head-injured college student. We have no information on such basic data as to how many college students have a head injury, how many head-injured students complete college, and how many head-injured individuals ultimately withdraw from college. Although Rimel and Jane (1983) reported that 24 percent of their sample of patients at a university hospital head-injury service were students, they did not specify if they were college level. Hall and De Pompei (1986) presented an article discussing some of the difficulties faced by head-injured college students. Bolger (1983) presented some common sequelae of head injuries but the article was not specifically related to the college setting.

It is clear that research is needed about the problems head-injured students face and ways to help with those problems. Any college professor, counselor or administrator can relate a number of cases of head-injured college students who were successful, or who simply disappeared from college life. What those personnel cannot tell is why the students withdrew, what kinds of problems the students faced, what helped the head-injured students, and how well the students were advised. There is no research about these matters.

The lack of information is in itself troubling, but the ramifications are even more so. The lack of empirical data on head-injured students means that potential college students (those in high school) and those already in college or returning to college after a head injury are being advised with virtually no factual information as the basis for that advice. The typical college professor, counselor or administrator (and, it must be noted, high school staff) does not have a great deal of knowledge of the effects of head injuries. What most professionals, including the majority of mental health workers such as psychologists, do not understand are the sometimes subtle yet serious cognitive (thinking) and behavioral effects of head injuries. This leads to such possibilities as the head-injured college student being advised to major in an academic area that is clearly inappropriate because of the nature of the head injury. It leads to students taking courses that will be unnecessarily frustrating, and attempting social situations that will lead to disappointment. These comments are not a criticism of the advisor or counselor; after all, one can only do as good a job as the available material permits, and much of that material is not yet available.

The lack of information further leads the college community to fail to recognize the head-injured student as needing any kind of special services (unless the student has obvious physical impairments), assuming such services are available. There are some programs specifically directed to the head-injured college student, one of the best known being the

California community colleges project described in detail in Cook (1987). Hackler and Tobis (1983) also described a community college project. The goals of these programs depend on the needs of the individual students, but range from independent community living to eventual entry by the student into a regular college curriculum. Unfortunately, most colleges and universities do not have programs that address the needs of the head-injured student who is taking regular classes at a school offering no special services for the head-injured person (or the person is not recognized as needing those services if they are available). I can immediately note such students from undergraduates to doctoral students.

Based on my personal experience, I continue to be amazed at the number of college students who casually indicate they have had brain injuries from any number of causes. These students are in the main stream of college life. They are seeking no special services and are not known to need them. During one semester alone I informally learned of six head-injured college students at my university, only two of whom were known by college personnel to be head injured (the students had not indicated the head injury to be a problem). Each of the students conveyed some kind of academically related problem as a result of the head injury. This book is written about and for those students.

CHAPTER 2

BRAIN ORGANIZATION AND THE EFFECTS OF HEAD INJURY

THE READER of this book need not have a detailed knowledge of brain anatomy, but it is helpful to have a general understanding of brain functioning and how impairments affect thinking and behavior. Advising the head-injured college student requires that one know the cognitive (thinking and intellectual functions), psychological, and social effects of head injuries, not the underlying physical bases of those behaviors. Knowing the relationship between brain areas and various abilities will, however, sharpen a person's understanding of the student. If nothing else, the knowledge is a way of establishing credibility with the student by being able to intelligently converse about the head injury. If uncertainties arise about an injury and its effects, there are excellent sources one may employ for more comprehensive information (Golden, 1981; Kolb & Whishaw, 1986).

BRAIN ORGANIZATION

In the early days of modern neurology one of the most widely debated topics was how specifically brain functions are located. Some anatomists believed that specific brain areas controlled specific mental functions or behaviors. This was called the localizationist argument. On the other hand, some believed the brain operated generally, as a total organ, with little or no specific control allotted to defined brain areas. For the interested reader, Valenstein (1973) presented an excellent history of this debate, but further discussion here is not necessary. The most prevalent view today of brain functioning is the one most eloquently presented by the late Russian neurologist and neuropsychologist, A. R.

Luria (1966, 1973). Luria viewed the brain as an interacting organ best thought of in terms of systems rather than discrete areas of functions. By this, Luria meant that various functions such as speech or movement actually involved a number of interconnected brain areas. For example, while we often refer to a speech center in the lower left frontal area of the brain called Broca's area (Broca was a French neurologist during the last century), this is not completely accurate. Broca's area controls only one aspect of the complex act of speaking, namely the process of converting ideas into spoken words. The physical ability to form words is governed by the motor strip (the precentral gyrus), which is near Broca's area but separate from it. The ability to form the ideas that will eventually become words depends on another area of the brain in and around a region called Wernicke's area, toward the back of the brain. Wernicke's area is connected to Broca's area by a bundle of nerve fibers technically called the arcuate fasiculus. Of course, all of these functions are dependent on the accurate reception and processing of impulses, seeing and hearing, for example, which are located in yet other areas of the brain. Disruption of any of these areas could result in a problem with speech. It is readily apparent that it is best to think of the brain as interconnected regions that form systems.

ESSENTIAL BRAIN ANATOMY

The brain is a rather small organ, given its immense importance. It weighs about three pounds and would almost fit in a man's cupped hands. Contrary to the popular perception, the brain is not a firm mass. It has the consistency of firm gelatin. Preparing a brain for anatomical study is actually a rather involved, time consuming process (Gluhbegovic & Williams, 1980). The purpose of this description is to lead to a very important point about head injuries. The brain is an extremely fragile, delicate organ consisting of billions of interconnecting fibers with less consistency than a strand of spider's web. Realizing this, it is not difficult to understand why even minor blows to the head present the potential for serious damage.

To protect the brain from external harm, it is encased in the skull, is surrounded by various protective membranes (the meninges) that help hold it in place, and is bathed in cerebrospinal fluid. This important fluid is produced within the brain's ventricles (four fluid filled spaces within the brain) and from there leaves the inside of the brain to surround the spinal cord and the space between the brain and the skull. It is not incorrect to think of the brain as floating in this fluid (with certain anchoring points, of course). The cerebrospinal fluid serves many purposes, but one of its most important is to cushion the brain from hitting the unyielding skull when a blow occurs. Unfortunately, the orbital base of the skull (above the eyes) contains bony ridges that can create serious damage when the brain is thrown against them. The cerebrospinal fluid is of limited value in protecting the brain in this region of the skull. By comparison, the back of the skull is relatively smooth.

A rich supply of blood with its nutrients and oxygen is needed to meet the intense metabolic requirements of the brain. Brain functioning can be maintained for only a few minutes if the blood supply is cut off. If the blood supply is diminished or cut off too long, death or permanent injury will result. The most well known example of a cut off of blood supply is a stroke. To insure proper blood flow, each side of the brain has its own blood supply, and there are blood-supply connections between the two sides.

The brain is an expansion of the spinal cord as the cord enters the skull or cranial vault. Upon entering the skull the spinal cord, carrying nerve impulses into the brain and back to the body, enlarges into various structures that ultimately become the cerebral hemispheres or brain as we usually think of it.

Just after entering the skull, the spinal cord enlarges into many structures (for example, the pons and medulla) that are generally collectively called the brainstem area. If one took a side view of the brain, the brainstem would be seen to extend into the middle part of the brain with a vast number of connecting fibers fanning out to all areas of the brain. Many of these fibers eventually end up at the cortex, the outer one-quarter inch of the brain that we recognize as the folded, convoluted part with its ridges (gyri, gyrus if singular) and the valleys between the ridges (sulci, sulcus if singular). Fiber tracts go back down to the spinal cord, making innumerable connections with other tracts and brain areas along the way.

The brainstem area controls basic life functions such as breathing, temperature control and heart rate. A particular structure of the brainstem known as the reticular formation is involved in how alert a person is to his or her environment. Damage to the brainstem area is often, but not always, fatal.

Behind the brainstem, that is toward the back of the head, is the cerebellum which looks like a miniature brain. It is intimately interconnected with the brainstem and higher areas on into the cortex. The cerebellum works with other brain areas to help coordinate motor movements, especially fine motor skills. Damage here will usually be evident in the person's impaired motor coordination.

The brain is a bilateral organ (two sides). Although we usually speak in the singular, for example, *the* hypothalamus, actually we should speak in the plural. There are two of everything in the brain, one on each side. This bilateral representation holds true with only an occasional exception. Although not a completely separate division, the right side of the body is controlled by the left side of the brain (left hemisphere) and the left side of the body is controlled by the right hemisphere. This is called contralateral control. Ipsilateral means on the same side. For example, impulses from the right ear go mainly to the left side of the brain (contralateral) but some go to the right side (ipsilateral). The general fact of contralateral control allows us to make a preliminary assessment of brain impairment. If the right side of the body is paralyzed, for example, we know the left side of the brain is damaged. This also allows us to make judgments about possible cognitive, social and behavioral difficulties, as these are also influenced by different sides of the brain in predictable ways.

The two hemispheres of the brain are not mirror images of themselves, whether in terms of physical qualities or in terms of function. These physical differences are not readily apparent, though. The work of many researchers, most notably Sperry (1974) has shown that the two hemispheres have different functions. Before going on, though, it is very important to realize that the two sides of the brain are not separate from each other. They are connected by many nerve fiber tracts called commisures, the largest of which is the corpus callosum. The corpus callosum runs roughly from the front of the brain to the back, along the upper part of the brain. The fibers making up this commisure radiate from all over one side of the brain and pass to the other side, carrying messages back and forth. The two sides of the brain are in instantaneous communication with each other. We do not have two brains within our skull. While the reader may have heard of the split-brain technique, a surgical procedure used to help control serious seizure disorders by severing varying degrees of the corpus callosum, many connecting tracts remain intact, and the brain is certainly not split. Research from split-brain humans and animals has shown the differences between functions of the right and left hemispheres (Sperry, 1974). For a more detailed discussion of the left and right hemisphere differences, Springer and

Deutsch (1985) is recommended, but an overview of these differences will be presented here.

The Left Hemisphere

The left side of the brain has traditionally been called the dominant hemisphere, not for any really justifiable reason, but simply because speech is usually located there, most people are right handed (left-side control), and the functions of the right hemisphere were not as well known. Because the areas for speech are usually located on the left side, this is often called the verbal hemisphere. The left hemisphere is considered to be logical, analytic and concerned with detail. Verbal analysis, mathematical abilities and verbal comprehension are left-side functions. Of course, motor control and sense perceptions on the right side of the body are controlled by the left hemisphere. Damage to the left hemisphere, depending of course on where it is, is likely to create motor or sensory problems on the right side of the body, speech difficulties, and some degree of word-handling (verbal) difficulty. Although not true in every case, often people with left hemisphere damage become anxious and depressed because they are aware of their newly acquired impairments. This is termed the catastrophic reaction.

The Right Hemisphere

The right side of the brain was once considered the silent or minor hemisphere. We now know that it is just as important as the left side of the brain and, in its own way, may be considered dominant for some functions. Until recently, the right hemisphere was thought of as nonverbal. The work of Sperry (1974), among others, has now shown that the right hemisphere does have verbal capacity. It can recognize speech and can form speech to some degree.

The right hemisphere controls motor and sensory functions on the left side of the body. It is thought of as the more emotional side which tends to look at situations on a more global or holistic scale than the left side. The right hemisphere pays less attention to detail than the left. Spatial abilities are mainly localized to the right hemisphere. Spatial ability refers to knowing where objects are (up, down, left, right, over, under, for example). This can be physical or mental (for example, keeping a column of numbers straight in one's head). Musical ability, at least the nonverbal part, is mainly right-side controlled. The word part of music belongs to the left hemisphere.

A peculiar effect of right hemisphere impairment is that the person may show a denial of damage and impairment in spite of obvious problems. To a lesser degree, there may be diminished recognition of the impairments. This is sometimes accompanied by an almost cheerful attitude. Technically, this is called anosognosia.

In general, damage to the right hemisphere will cause spatial problems, failure to grasp the overall picture of something while understanding details, and difficulties dealing with emotional situations. Of course, left-side motor and sensory difficulties would be expected with right-side damage.

It cannot be overemphasized that the two hemispheres of the brain work in conjunction with each other, not independently. For the most part, the left-right differences described here are not noticeable because the brain is acting as a total organ, not as two sides free of each other's control. The differences are important in understanding brain function.

The Lobes of the Brain

Each hemisphere of the brain is divided into four lobes or areas that are not easily demarcated and are not readily apparent when one views a brain or a photograph of one. The term lobe gives the impression that there are four discrete areas that could be lifted out and separated. In reality, we are referring to the outer layer of the brain—the cortex. When a surgeon speaks of removing a lobe, it usually means removal of the cortex only. The rest of the brain, that below the cortex, is called subcortical, and consists of the ventricles (discussed earlier in this chapter), billions of connecting nerve fibers between cortical areas, cortical and subcortical areas (including the brainstem), and subcortical to subcortical areas. There are specific bundles of fibers called nuclei that relate to functions such as memory, motor control, and emotions. The terms grey matter and white matter refer to the appearance of the neurons and neuronal tracts. If the tract is covered with a white, fatty substance called myelin, it is called white matter. Other neuronal matter is called grey matter, for example, the cortex, because it lacks myelination.

The Occipital Lobes. The occipital lobes (remember, there is one on each side) are located at the very back of the brain toward the bottom. It is here that impulses, running along nerve tracts from the eyes and through the brain, are received and translated into something recognizable. The occipital lobes are the most restricted of the four lobes in terms of function in that they serve one main function: visual reception and analysis. Obviously, any damage along the nerve tracts or in the occipital region will result in some degree of visual disturbance from blindness to restricted vision to the failure to recognize an object even though the eyes are working properly. An interesting dysfunction (*dys* means impaired) is called visual neglect. In this problem, the person does not attend to some part of the visual field. For example, with left-field visual neglect the person sees only the right half of a picture or reads only the right half of a sentence. It is remarkable that the person is often unaware of the problem and must be taught to compensate for the dysfunction by turning his or her head to complete the visual field.

The Parietal Lobes. These lobes cover roughly the back one-third of the brain. They begin at the central sulcus, a landmark of the brain more or less in line with your ear upward, and go back to meet the occipital lobes and the back of the temporal lobes. The divisions between these lobes are not clear or readily apparent.

The parietal lobes receive incoming tactual (feeling) sensations from the opposite side of the body. These impulses end in what is called the sensory strip, or post-central gyrus (the first gyrus after the central sulcus). The incoming impulses are interpreted in the area next to where they are received. These lobes, then, let the person know he or she has been touched or has touched something, and the details of that sensation (light, heavy, location, for example).

Spatial abilities are also controlled mainly by the parietal lobes, more so on the right than on the left. The left parietal lobe, being on the verbal side of the brain for most people, has a great deal to do with verbal analysis (understanding words and their relationship to each other) and mathematical abilities. The parietal lobes also help direct behavior in that physical movements are dependent on signals from sensory sensations, such as where one foot is in relation to the other, or where the left hand is in relation to the right.

Impairment in the parietal lobes, depending on the specific location of damage, may interfere with physical feeling and the ability to know what has been touched on the opposite side of the body. Motor performance may be impaired because of disturbed sensory feedback. Spatial difficulties are likely, which has special ramifications for the college student. He or she will experience difficulty keeping in mind where buildings are in relation to each other. Some academic areas are especially dependent on spatial abilities, physical and mental. Specifically, there may be problems in subjects requiring keeping numbers in proper spatial relationship such as borrowing in subtraction or keeping a column of numbers in proper order during addition. Academic areas such as art, architecture, geometry, and engineering may well present problems related to impaired spatial abilities. By now it has undoubtedly been noted that the word *may* is being overused. This is intentional because we lack the empirical evidence to verify these suggestions. At this point, caution is advisable.

The Temporal Lobes. The temporal lobes are located along the outer, bottom part of the brain, corresponding to an area above your ear and somewhat toward the front. At the back, they blend in with the occipital lobes and the bottom of the parietal lobes. The temporal lobes have complex functions. They are the receiving sites for incoming auditory sensations from both the contralateral and the ipsilateral ear. The part of the brain that comprehends speech is at the upper back part of the left temporal lobe in most people, in a region known as Wernicke's area. The ideas for speech are formed in this region of the brain and are ultimately sent to the frontal lobes to be converted to speech.

Going from the temporal cortex in toward the middle part of the brain, the brainstem area, are some extremely important subcortical structures often described as deep within the temporal lobes. The hippocampus is a structure near the brainstem that begins the memory process, once an event has occurred to be remembered. The hippocampus begins the encoding (storage) process of memory. From the hippocampus, memory is apparently sent all over the cortex for storage, a process not yet well understood. Without the hippocampi (there are two, one on each side) memory would be impossible. With bilateral (both sides) destruction of the hippocampi, no new memories could be stored, but memories stored before the damage would remain intact. A person could recall a childhood event but not remember the name of a person he or she just met. Damage to one hippocampus does not create such a serious dysfunction because the other hippocampus, which is connected to the damaged one, continues to function.

Also deep within the temporal lobes, around the brainstem area is the limbic system, a combination of brain structures that is variously described by different authors. One writer may include a structure that another writer does not include in the limbic system. The limbic system has significant connections with the frontal lobes, more specifically with what is called the prefrontal area. These connections are most important in reference to the control of emotions, but more will be said about this in the next section. For now, it is important to note that the limbic system relates to what is generally called motivation and emotions. The bases for such drives as anger, fear, thirst, hunger, and emotions are centered in the limbic system. To some degree, sexual drives are also located here.

Damage to the temporal lobes may create a variety of impairments. Hearing may be impaired, but it will be recalled that hearing from each ear is represented on both sides of the brain. Damage to one temporal lobe will not totally destroy hearing. A more likely problem related to hearing is difficulty discriminating sounds from each other. This makes understanding other people more difficult because the sound of their voice is not as clearly discriminated as it should be. Damage to Wernicke's area creates a disorder known as Wernicke's aphasia. In this disorder, the ears are unimpaired, hearing is quite adequate, but what is being heard makes no sense (just as you would feel if someone spoke to you in a language you did not understand; your ears would hear the sounds but the sounds would mean nothing to you). In Wernicke's aphasia the person has fluent speech but it is for the most part meaningless. The listener cannot understand what is being said. Also, with Wernicke's aphasia, the patient cannot repeat what has been said to him or her.

Damage to the limbic system creates the potential for difficulty with emotional reactions ranging from relatively unemotional to overly emotionally reactive. The emotional reactions of others may be misunderstood. Memory impairment is likely with temporal lobe damage.

Head injury involving the temporal lobes relates to the college student in a more general way than it does to specific academic areas. Clearly, if memory is significantly impaired, all aspects of college will be difficult if not impossible. Emotional reactions may create difficulties in social situations. With Wernicke's aphasia, college is not likely to be a viable alternative because of the comprehension, verbal expression, and written expression that are required to go through college. Any subject that requires discrimination of sounds such as music or foreign languages may be expected to present problems. One might surmise that music would be more affected by right temporal damage, while foreign languages would be more affected by left-side difficulties.

The Frontal Lobes. The frontal lobes start at the central sulcus (the landmark running upward, roughly above the ears) and continue forward to above the eyes. The parietal and frontal lobes meet at the central sulcus. The very front of the frontal lobes, just above the eyes, is called the prefrontal or far frontal area. At the back of the frontal lobes, along the central sulcus, is the motor strip (precentral gyrus), running from the temporal lobe at the bottom, up to the top of the brain where the cortex turns downward on itself in the middle, down toward the brainstem. The motor strip, along with some subcortical areas (for example, what are called the basal ganglia) and the cerebellum control physical movements on the opposite side of the body. The signals move from the motor strip down along various pathways (e.g., the internal capsule) to the spinal cord and on to the body. In front of the motor strip, toward the front of the head, is where physical movements are organized into recognizable patterns such as picking up an object or carrying out a series of movements. These movement patterns are stored in this area of the brain.

The prefrontal region, just above the eyes, is the part of the brain that controls social behavior and personality. It is here that people plan, organize their lives, devise plans to carry out actions, exert judgment, and make assessments of the appropriateness of their actions. Due to the interconnections with the limbic system, the prefrontal area exerts what we call social control over the basic drives and emotions. It is this part of the brain that keeps our behavior socially appropriate. Without it, human actions would more closely resemble animal behaviors.

A critical area of the left frontal lobe (for most people) is an area just in front of the motor strip but separate from it, and above the temporal lobe. This is Broca's area, where the ideas for speech are actually translated into verbal expression (words). Damage here results in Broca's aphasia, a disorder in which the person can understand speech, can form the ideas of speech, but cannot form the words for verbal expression. The person knows what he or she wants to say, but the words do not come out right. Speech is limited in terms of speed and available words, with speech often being slow and telegraphic in style. With lesser degrees of damage, of course, the amount of verbal output may increase to where speech is obviously impaired but understandable.

Damage to the motor strip results in impaired physical movements on the opposite side of the body (in degrees, of course), corresponding to the affected area of the motor strip. If damage occurs in the region adjacent to the motor strip, toward the front, the person's ability to carry out the proper sequence of physical actions will be impaired. In terms of college, it is apparent that any subject requiring physical skills will be more difficult for the impaired person than the person with intact motor abilities. Difficulty would be expected in such subjects as woodworking, art, playing a musical instrument, or physical education. Simply stated, there must be correspondence between the physical ability of the head-injured person and the physical requirements of a task. Careful assessment must be made of potentially dangerous situations such as working around machines or electricity, or working with dangerous chemicals.

It is damage to the prefrontal region that presents the most perplexing and frequently misunderstood impairments. We must remind ourselves that the ability to plan, organize, follow through with plans, exert good judgment, show social restraint, and realize the effect of our actions on others are brain functions that can be, and are, impaired just as surely as vision, sensation, or physical movements can be impaired by brain injury. Damage to the prefrontal region and its connections with the limbic system may result in poor judgment, impulsivity, lowered social restraint, emotional reactions, and impaired planning and organizing abilities. The person with prefrontal damage may appear to others as irresponsible and unreliable. The head-injured person does not follow through with necessary plans and promised actions, even very important ones such as enrollment or keeping a social engagement. The person seems to lack an overall plan for where he or she is going in life, even though at the moment very good plans may be presented by the person. In extreme cases the person may appear unusually unmotivated and unresponsive to his or her environment. Uncharacteristic unsociable behavior may emerge because the controls from the prefrontal region to the limbic system are lacking. There may be problems of emotional control due to limbic system damage.

Given the social and personality control allotted to the frontal lobes, it is unfortunate that they rest in a region of the skull with bony ridges at the base. It is almost assured that irrespective of where a blow to the head occurs, the frontal, especially prefrontal, areas of the brain will be affected as they come in contact with these ridges. The very front of the temporal lobes are also likely to incur damage for the same reason. Thus, just about any blow to the head, if serious enough, will result in prefrontal and temporal lobe damage which, in turn, creates a cluster of symptoms that are not likely to be seen by most people as brain related.

The impairment of social and personality skills have a direct impact on college life in a most pervasive way. The ability to get through courses and through college in general requires a great deal of planning, organizing, judgment, social awareness, and personal awareness.

The Association Areas. The interacting brain, discussed earlier, can be exemplified by describing the areas where the various lobes come together and overlap. For example, where the parietal, temporal, and occipital lobes converge toward the back of the brain is an area called the angular gyrus. On the left side of the brain this is the region where a word that is read begins its journey into action. The word is seen and read (occipital lobe for vision and parietal lobe for proper spatial sequence of the letters). The word is then recognized and called up from memory to be given meaning (temporal lobe). The visual, spatial and memory aspects are joined in the angular gyrus from which the word is sent to the frontal lobes for a proper response (running, if the word happens to be *danger*). Of course, the two sides of the brain are in constant interaction throughout the process.

Throughout the brain are multitudes of such association and integration areas. To understand a person's impairments we must move beyond a lobe-by-lobe account of damage in which we try to simply add the effects to each other. We must analyze the person in terms of the dynamic interplay of brain systems.

INDIVIDUAL DIFFERENCES

Because the brain is a dynamic, interacting organ, even small degrees of damage may have profound effects on other regions of the brain. Since every person is unique, and every brain is unique, it is not possible to make one-to-one comparisons between brain damage and behavior from person to person. The picture is much too complex to allow this. Each person must be understood individually, a point I cannot overemphasize. Two people with apparently the same degree of damage in the same region of the brain may present two completely different configurations of impairments and preserved abilities. The differences are due to the uniqueness of the brains, personality traits of the person before and after the damage, and the day to day situation the person lives in. As an example, assume two people with right parietal lobe damage are injured to the same degree. The first person, recognizing the spatial difficulties resulting from the injury, lives on campus, with a clear set of daily instructions, and a set pattern of going from one place to another (or at least a clear map of the campus suitably altered to address the spatial difficulty, for example, color coded). His or her environment is stable, predictable, and structured. This person is adjusting well. The second person lives in a large apartment complex many blocks from campus, having to pass through a very busy business district to get to campus. There are numerous opportunities for spatial problems to arise, and they undoubtedly will. This person is tense, anxious, depressed, and easily distracted. This person is not adjusting well. The differences are not due to brain injury per se, but to the differences in living arrangements. Understanding the individual requires an analysis of the overall situation, not just the brain injury itself.

THE SPECIAL CASE OF THE CLOSED HEAD INJURY

Closed head injuries (CHI) mean the head has received a blow but the skull was not penetrated or broken through. The most common cause of closed head injuries is automobile accidents, but any other type of blow to the head may result in a closed head injury. An especially tragic form of closed head injury results from an infant or young child being violently shaken, causing the brain to repeatedly hit the skull as it moves back and forth and around the brain stem.

In contrast to the closed head injury, a penetrating wound is where the skull was broken through. A penetrating wound is usually recognized to be a brain problem because there are visible signs of entry (scarring, indentions). Of course, a closed head injury may also present such visible signs as well as obvious physical symptoms such as paralysis. These cases of closed head injury are also recognized as having a brain injury.

There are, however, a large but unspecified number of closed head injuries that do not present any noticeable indications of damage or clear-cut physical symptoms. These people are not likely to be recognized as being head-injured. In Chapter 1 the effects of even minor head injuries were discussed, many of which would not be recognized as having any residual brain disorder. Even serious brain injury may present no obvious, observable signs of impairment. The person with such injuries will very likely go unrecognized as permanently injured, and may not even be aware of the problems himself or herself. Even sophisticated brain imaging techniques such as the CT scan or Magnetic Resonance Imaging (MRI, a technique something like a CT but with a clearer image) may miss the damage.

The lack of observable impairment is deceptive. In closed head injuries genuine brain impairment may go unrecognized, but the problems are just as real as demonstrable physical symptoms. The damage in closed head injuries comes from two major sources: the brain hitting the skull in general, but especially the skull region above the eyes; and a process called axonal shearing (axons are part of the nerve cells, neurons, that make up the message-carrying fibers). When a person's head hits something, or is hit by something, the brain is thrown against the skull. The damage at the point of impact is called the coup injury (coup means blow). However, as the brain moves from the impact it is thrown against the opposite skull, resulting in contrecoup injury, injury opposite the point of impact. A person could receive a blow to the left temporal region (coup injury) but, because the brain is thrown against the right skull, have more severe damage on the right side (contrecoup injury) than the left.

Regardless of the point of impact, the frontal lobes and frontal pole (tip) of the temporal lobes are likely to be damaged in a closed head injury. Thus, a blow from the back of the head, side of the head, or from the front is very likely to result in frontal and temporal lobe injury as the lobes strike the bony ridges in the orbital part of the skull. This is an important point to remember because a person is likely to show symptoms of frontal lobe damage even though the frontal area was not directly involved in the impact.

Axonal shearing refers to the severing of nerve pathways within the brain. In a closed head injury the brain is not only thrown back and forth, it also twists around the brainstem (torque). Remembering that the brain has the consistency of gelatin and that there are billions of web-thin fibers connecting areas of the brain, it is not difficult to imagine the damage from even a minor impact.

The shearing of the neuronal pathways means the brain is not as able as it once was to effectively communicate within itself. It cannot efficiently send the necessary messages it must send to effect a well-functioning person. Quite simply, the system has been irreparably interrupted, with the amount of disruption depending upon the amount of axonal shearing and where the shearing took place. Since no two accidents are the same, no two people will have exactly the same degrees and location of shearing.

As was noted previously, it is virtually certain that a closed head injury will result in some degree of impairment in the frontal lobes and frontal-limbic connections. Add to the injury picture any other problems resulting from coup and contrecoup damage and the symptom picture becomes complex. Neuropsychological testing of closed-head-injured persons often shows an overall lowering of cognitive functioning, but with some functions well preserved and others seriously impaired (depending on the degree of injury, of course).

It is clear that a closed head injury without obvious physical signs presents a serious potential for misunderstanding by other people, and, perhaps, by the injured person himself or herself. Imagine having the ability to plan behaviors in proper sequence, carry through with intentions, organize life, maintain social awareness, and understand the reactions of others suddenly dissolve and not realize it is a brain problem. Even worse, imagine how the closed-head-injured person feels when friends, family, employers or professors suggest he or she is thoughtless or irresponsible.

For those seeking a greater understanding of closed head injuries, many sources are available. The book by Levin, Benton, and Grossman (1982) is an especially good source on this topic.

RECOVERY AND REHABILITATION

A comprehensive discussion of recovery and rehabilitation is beyond the scope of this book. By the time the head-injured person reaches college he or she will have completed a rehabilitation program or will be in one (assuming the head injury was recognized and treated, an assumption that is debatable in some cases). Nonetheless, a brief discussion of recovery and rehabilitation will help better prepare the reader to advise the head-injured college student.

The possibility of recovery from brain injury has dramatically improved in recent times (Begali, 1987). The change is due to more rapid and sophisticated medical treatment (Hackler & Tobis, 1983). Whether the person resumes a normal pre-injury life depends on the degree of residual physical impairments, remaining cognitive abilities, psychological adjustment, and the amount of emotional and social support the person will have after recovery.

Two of the most important predictors of recovery from a brain injury are the length of time in a coma and the length of blank time between the injury and the recovery of memory (called the PTA, post-traumatic amnesia time). See Plum and Posner (1982) and Victors and Adams (1985) for further discussion of these important measures, but for now it is adequate to note that generally the longer these two measures are the less likely the person will be able to resume a normal pre-injury life. The data are very clear that the longer these two measures, for as short as a few days in a coma, the lower the likelihood of complete post-injury recovery. The relationship between these two measures and the outcome of an injury is rather easy to understand: the longer the coma or PTA, the greater amount of damage it took to produce them.

The age of the person at the time of the injury is a factor in recovery. Generally, the younger the person at the time of injury, the greater the chance for a full or nearly full recovery (Miller, 1984). Although there is some debate about the validity of the concept, the idea that a young brain is more amenable to recovery is called brain plasticity. This means that the younger the brain, the greater the probability that some other area of the brain will take over the functions of the damaged area. With or without the concept of plasticity, it is valid to say that the older the person at the time of injury, the less likely he or she is to fully recover.

Recovery from brain injury, if serious, may require long hospitalization followed by rehabilitation in such areas as speech therapy, physical therapy, occupational therapy, cognitive retraining, and memory retraining. Social skills training, as well as personal counseling may be necessary as the person re-enters the community. Brain-injury rehabilitation presents remarkably ingenious ways to help the person regain skills or find ways to compensate for them. Among many books, the ones by Golden (1981), Ylvisaker (1985), and Meier, Benton, and Dillers (1987) give a good presentation of some of these remarkable techniques.

For the person working with the head-injured college student, several points must be kept in mind. Recovery from a head-injury may be quite rapid or may take several years, although for most people the greatest amount of recovery will occur within the first few months of the injury (Jennett, 1983a). The prospective student should take these points into consideration and not rush back to school or begin it for the first time too soon after the injury. Recall that Rimel, Giordini, Barth, Boll, and Jane (1981) found even minor head injuries had repercussions lasting several months post-injury. The student may create a frustrating failure experience by attempting college too soon. The student may begin to feel depressed, discouraged, and anxious, resulting in withdrawal from school. Had the person waited, some of these concerns may have been avoided.

A FINAL NOTE: EXPECT THE UNEXPECTED

One topic remains to close this chapter: the sometimes bewildering ways brain impairments and preserved functions show themselves. At times, what appears to be inexplicable variations in performance of the head-injured person leave the impression that the person is manipulating the symptoms to his or her advantage. The head-injured person who usually shows poor judgment exhibits uncharacteristically good judgment in some situation. A person with poor memory shows remarkable recall for something that was promised, or where something was stored. The individual who generally seems inattentive, detects a detail missed by others. The person who sits quietly, noting overwhelming fatigue that prevents completion of a necessary task responds with energy and enthusiasm at the suggestion of going out for the evening.

One of the first patients I observed as a postdoctoral intern in neuropsychology was a man interviewed by my supervisor. The man suffered Broca's aphasia and could use only one word in responding to questions, which he clearly understood. The patient would use this single word over and over in responding. After many minutes of this, he was asked to repeat a five-word phrase. He repeated it flawlessly. The part of the brain that controls initiation of speech was impaired, but the part that controls repetition was not.

I twice tested a patient with severe right frontal damage and less severe left frontal and parietal damage. He had an obvious scar running across the top of his head from temple to temple, the result of surgery. At the first testing, three weeks post-injury, I was informed by the client that he had fallen in the shower and that was how he got the scar. At the second testing, eight weeks post-injury, he informed me he had fallen on the sidewalk. Even after I provided details of the injury and surgery, he pleasantly denied ever having been injured or having had surgery. This was not a psychological denial, it is a brain-related disorder termed anosognosia.

In each of these examples and many more that could have been used, the head-injured person was not in any way being consciously manipulative. The person was reflecting the effects of the injury and preserved functions. These were not "psychological" problems. Although it may tax one's ability to understand *how* brain injury can create these problems, to help the head-injured person it must be accepted that these are related to physical causes, not mental or psychological difficulties.

CHAPTER 3

IS COLLEGE A VIABLE ALTERNATIVE?

GIVEN THE descriptions presented in the previous chapter, it is legitimate to ask if the head-injured person should even try college for the first time or return to it after a head injury. The answer to the question is that many head-injured people do go on to college and do graduate. Obviously, the decision to attempt college must be made on an individual basis, not on the basis of general suggestions. For some head-injured individuals college would be a devastating experience, while for others it would be an enjoyable, rewarding one.

College is certainly not for everyone, head-injured or not. There are many pathways to a happy, fulfilling life, and college is only one of those ways. For some people, college is a necessity because of the profession they have chosen, teaching, medicine, or psychology, for example. For these people, college is a demanding time but this is countered by the recognition that all the work is in the interest of achieving a worthwhile goal. For other people, going to college has no specific career meaning; rather, it is seen as a demanding but enjoyable experience of being exposed to new areas of knowledge. The goal here is more personal fulfillment than vocational. For the third group, college has no immediate purpose in terms of personal or vocational goals. This person is in college for a variety of reasons other than really wanting to be there. Their reasons for attending college may include parental expectations, peer pressure, or the perception that there are no good alternatives. Under these conditions college will be tolerated, at best, and will be a source of frustration and disappointment, at worst. It is advisable for this person to not attempt college until he or she is ready for it. The fourth group of people are those for whom college would be too difficult because of their psychological condition or because of the intellectual demands placed on them. Whether congenital or acquired, the intellectual inability to complete college clearly indicates that college is not a viable alternative (if the problem is a psychological one, therapy is likely to help). In the case of the brain-injured person, if cognitive abilities are so impaired as to prevent effective functioning (for example, extremely poor memory or significantly impaired comprehension) it would be unnecessarily stressful to even encourage college attendance. There are other ways for this person to find a fulfilling life.

Simply stated, are we setting up the head-injured person for failure if we encourage going to college? Are we expecting too much of the person, given his or her newly acquired impairments? Again, as I noted earlier in this chapter, these are not unrealistic goals if the person has the ability to do it and especially the motivation to go to college. Skill and intelligence alone are not enough to successfully complete college. It takes dedication. It takes the willingness to delay other attractive goals. All these points must be considered when helping a person decide about college.

INTELLECTUAL FUNCTIONING IN THE HEAD-INJURED

A discussion of intelligence would be a most lengthy aside to this book. There is no uniform agreement as to what intelligence is and what contributes to it. While most people have a relatively useful idea about intelligence, the academic study of it can be very deep and can raise question after question. Without further discussion of the various theories of intelligence, I will refer the reader to a most interesting book on this topic in which the idea of different kinds of intelligence is discussed (Gardner, 1983).

There is no single area of the brain where intelligence is located. All areas of the brain contribute to the general function of intelligence. This presents two important points. First, since intelligence is not restricted to any specific part of the brain, just about any injury will have some effect on intellectual functioning (e.g., perception, memory, mathematical ability, verbal reasoning). The specific deficits may be readily apparent or of only minor significance. The second point is that irrespective of degree of injury, some aspect of intellectual functioning will remain. The head-injured person must capitalize on the remaining abilities.

Research and experience has shown that individuals with brain injuries, even serious ones, can produce normal test results on intelligence measures. Halstead (1947) noted that patients with serious frontal lobe damage could perform normally on tests of intelligence (if the tests were measuring global, rather than specific, abilities). This led to the belief that the frontal lobes were "silent," a point we now know to be untrue. Essentially, the problem with the earlier results was that researchers were not measuring the right skills with the right tests.

We must realize that to go to college, remain employed, or simply get along in life requires more than just being intellectually bright. The bright person must behave in an intelligent way; the intelligence must be *used* effectively. We can all think of people who are very bright, intellectually, but who do not function well in the everyday world because of emotional problems, lack of motivation, or, in the case of this book, head injury. Brain impairment may leave the person intellectually intact overall, but with subtle problems such as discrimination difficulties, impaired planning, slight memory loss, or problems in social control that could undermine a successful college experience. The fact that overall intellectual abilities remain grossly intact does not necessarily indicate success in college will be assured. Each person must have a thorough evaluation of intellectual abilities as part of deciding whether or not college is a viable alternative for that person. Certainly, college should not be categorically ruled out simply because a person has incurred a head injury.

TRANSITION TO THE VOCATIONAL SETTING

The decision that a head-injured person is capable of going to college does not end the decision process. An equally important question remains: whether or not the person will be able to effectively carry through with the demands of his or her chosen profession. It is common knowledge that going from the college setting to the vocational world is sometimes difficult. The transition from the academic world to the work setting requires adaptability and resourcefulness. A person can only rarely directly and concretely apply what was learned in the classroom to the demands of the job.

Even if the person has the necessary adaptability to make the transfer from classroom to workplace, other problems will present themselves. The demands of a job are daily, all day, not a few hours a day, two or three times a week as would be true in college. With difficulty handling such pressure, the job may quickly become overwhelming. The new college graduate will very likely find the vocational setting to be more demanding in terms of quantity of output and speed of performance. The employer is likely to be less tolerant of late assignments and having to make special accommodations for the head-injured person.

If the previous two paragraphs have left a slightly negative feeling, that was certainly not the intent. It is a matter of insuring that if employment is the goal of going to college, fulfilling employment can be found that is consistent with the person's abilities. It would be unfair to promote going to college if the person's goals cannot be reached. If our best judgment is that a person is going to face unusual problems, he or she must be informed of them. It is ultimately the head-injured person's decision to take the risks or avoid them, but it is the responsibility of the advisor to be sure the decision is an informed one.

Should the person decide not to pursue a given vocation, college is not necessarily ruled out. There are other vocational possibilities, subject to the same qualifications already noted.

SUCCESSFUL HEAD-INJURED COLLEGE STUDENTS

Success stories of head-injured college students are more frequent than people might imagine. It is not that the head-injured college students are not succeeding, it is simply that the success is not noted. In many cases, the person was not even known by others to be head-injured. Since many cases go unnoticed, the impression is left that there are not very many head-injured college students. Even as I am writing this book, I continue to be amazed by the number of people who, learning of this project, relate to me the story of a friend, relative, colleague or themselves who is (are) going to college and is doing well. Only occasionally is the head-injured person known to the college as being head-injured.

Virtually anyone working in the head-injury field can relate a number of stories about his or her clients who successfully went on to college or returned to college after an injury. Bauer and Titonis (1987), noting some of the difficulties faced by head-injured college students, nonetheless noted, "We have worked with head-injured young adults who have returned to college and successfully completed their course of studies" p. 407. Hebb (1939) noted the case of a patient with a very high level of intelligence who had undergone a pre-frontal lobectomy (removal of the lobe). This patient not only finished college, but he went on to do well in medical school. The recordings of various meetings addressing the needs of head-injured college students (Savage, Cohen, Coyne, Fryer, & Harrington, 1985; Cook, Knight, & Harrington, 1986; Cook & Knight, 1987; Holmes, 1987) attest to the presence of such students. My own preliminary research (Holmes, 1988) in which I surveyed rehabilitation facilities about clients going on to college indicates that somewhere around 20 per cent (on average) start or return to college. Somewhere around 60 per cent of these clients remained in college. These are very preliminary data. Future research may well indicate different figures, but for now the important message is that head-injured persons are going to college and are doing so in apparently large numbers.

Coming back to the original intent of this chapter, asking if college is a viable alternative for the head-injured individual, the answer is a qualified, "yes." If the strengths, impairments, needs, appropriateness of goals, and the personality and social abilities of the person are carefully considered, college can be a successful experience. As I noted earlier in this chapter, college is not appropriate for everyone, with or without head injury. One should not assume the head-injured person cannot go to college and we should not assume college is the appropriate goal for all head-injured people.

After the acute medical crises have passed and the person has had time to adjust to any acquired impairments, a careful consideration and evaluation of the person and the demands of college life will allow the best estimate of success. I cannot overemphasize that there is a great deal to be learned about the head-injured college student. As more is learned, the chances of success will increase as our decision process becomes more refined.

CHAPTER 4

COMMON PROBLEMS OF THE HEAD-INJURED COLLEGE STUDENT

AT THE RISK of being repetitive, I must again note that every head-injured person is first an individual. The person's personality, life situation, location and extent of damage, and ability to deal with the head injury combine to create the unique person. To discuss common problems is to discuss problems *most* people will face. On an individual by individual basis, any given person may or may not have the problems to be discussed in this chapter. It is wise to assume nothing about a person simply because he or she is head-injured. A complete assessment is necessary to effectively advise the person.

COMPARING COLLEGE AND HIGH SCHOOL

Given the large amount of material available on the head-injured student from preschool to high school, it is reasonable to ask why we cannot simply take that material and use it with the college student. We *can* use some of that information, of course. The cognitive problems from brain injury such as poor memory, impaired reasoning, or disorientation are just as applicable to college as they are to high school. However, some very real differences between college and high school present the potential for increased stress for the college student. To assume the head-injured high school student will automatically be able to make the transition to college is not a justifiable assumption. High school students without head injuries face difficult adjustments to college life, and one would expect no less from the head-injured person. In the following pages the eight significant differences between high school and college will be presented.

Structure. College is much less structured than high school. The typical high school follows a prescribed program over a set period of time, usually three or four years. The high school day starts at a regular time, ends at a regular time, and class follows class on some fairly stable schedule. Attendance is monitored by the school, and the students' whereabouts are routinely noted. High school meets daily, Monday through Friday.

College classes meet at various times, from early morning to evenings and weekends. They may range from one day a week to daily. A particular student may have one class a day, all classes on two or three days, or any other possible combination. Although the classes are regularly scheduled, they do not necessarily follow one another; in fact, there may be long periods of time between classes. Attendance may or may not be monitored, and no one keeps track of a student's whereabouts. Graduating from college may be in as few as two or three years or may stretch out over many years, depending on the student's abilities and desires.

College is clearly less structured than high school. This places a greater personal responsibility on the college student to attend classes, plan classes and overall goals to graduation, and get assignments completed on time. In college, it is assumed the student is mature and responsible enough to meet these demands.

Freedom to Choose. Although high schools do offer some choices of classes, they generally have a much more defined program than college. The high school student has limited choices about what classes to take and when to take them. The college student has a great deal more freedom to choose classes and schedules. Of course, college requires certain classes, but there is often a fairly large array of times offered for those classes, and the student may fit the class anywhere he or she wants in the college career. A class may be avoided for several semesters or may be taken immediately. It is not unusual for a college junior or senior to finally take a dreaded class that other students took their first semester.

The college student has much greater freedom to tailor a program to suit his or her needs, both in terms of time and interest. Various classes may be taken to fill an interest that is not formally offered by the college.

The freedom to choose in college, and the responsibility that goes along with it, is no more evident than in the college student having to declare a major area of study such as business or psychology. In high school the student does not major in specific areas; rather, a general education or college preparatory course is taken. In college the student is offered a sometimes bewildering number of possible major areas. Abilities, personal interests, and practical matters such as finances or eventually finding employment enter into the decision to major in a given academic area. The typical student has a number of possible areas in which he or she might major, but, unless more time is taken to graduate, only one of them can be chosen. It is not always easy to make these choices, but they must be made. The only alternative is to major in more than one area, which means more time in school, or to pursue a general studies program if the college has one.

Pace of Studies. Because high school must accomodate a wide variety of intellectual abilities and motivational levels, the pace of studies must be slower than it is in college. The high school student may read a few pages of assignments or complete an art project over a whole term. In that same time the college student may have read several chapters or even severals books, and will have completed an art project every week or two. The high school student may be allowed several days to write a theme that the college student is expected to write during a 50-minute class session. A term paper in high school, if required at all, may entail 5 to 10 pages with a few references. The college paper may be 20 to 30 pages long with detailed references. I certainly realize that I am generalizing, and that some high schools are quite demanding.

The college student is expected to do a great deal more work and to do it in less time than the high school student. At the graduate level, working on a master's or doctoral degree, the pace is significantly increased even compared to the undergraduate pace of studies.

Academic Expectations. Avoiding the debate about the current level of academic standards in high schools and colleges, I will note that as a general rule the academic expectations in college are greater. This is especially true as one progresses through college. For example, a sophomore class in college may require reading a 300-page book and taking four examinations (or more). The senior-level class may require reading a 600-page book and taking only two or three examinations. Beyond the sheer amount of work in college is the less tangible but equally important expectation that the quality of work must be higher than in high school. A theme that was given a high grade in high school may be seen as mediocre in college. A good psychology experiment in high school may be seen as unsophisticated at the college level. The leading role in a high school play may be seen as amateurish. What was acceptable in high school may not be acceptable in college.

Tolerance for Academic Disinterest. I am not implying that high schools encourage or appreciate disinterest in school, but high schools are generally forced to deal with more of it because the students constitute a forced audience. Either the law or parental demands require the student to attend classes, but neither can make the student become interested in the class. The high school student who is not interested in the class will do minimal work and is likely to be more interested in socializing than studying. In many cases, alternatives are limited, and this disinterested attitude must be tolerated.

At the college level, the student who consistently fails to attend class, is not attentive, and fails to keep up with assignments is likely to be dropped from the class or, at best, suffer a lowered grade. Expulsion from college is frequently required when a person's academic performance drops below a certain level. In high school such expulsion is less likely if the problem is purely an academic one. Even if the disinterested college student manages to stay in college, recommendations from the faculty will reflect the student's poor performance. Employment and graduate school are likely to be compromised when the recommendations are not positive.

Physical Facilities. With occasional exceptions, the high school is usually housed in a single building. The college is, with rare exception, almost never contained in a single building. The typical college campus covers many acres with many buildings. At a larger university it is not unusual for buildings to be several blocks apart, and in no particular system that would help the student keep them clearly in mind. Some college campuses are divided into two or more separate locations, sometimes relatively close to each other, and sometimes at a significant distance.

The typical college campus is much more complex, physically large, and widely scattered than the usual high school. The college student must often quickly shuttle from one building to another, and must, of course, keep a quick mental map of their locations.

Competitiveness. The new college student is likely to find himself or herself in a surprisingly competitive environment, especially in the upper-level courses. The majority of students in the class want to be there and really do want to learn. They will exert great effort to learn the subject matter of the course. The student who in high school was able to slip by with a casual comment about a subject will be among people who realize the superficiality of the response and who will not be the least bit reticent in pointing it out. The new college student is now perhaps with students who have gone to larger schools with a greater number of classes and experiences. Some of the fellow students were in advanced high school classes and are clearly better prepared than their classmates. This can lead to a threatening and discouraging situation, especially for the student from a very small high school where academic competition was limited.

Social Expectations. As any college student personnel worker can attest, first entering college is often a serious adjustment for most students. The college student is expected to be mature, self-directed, confident, and capable of analytic thought. All of this is expected a mere few weeks after leaving the high school in which the student was directed rather than self-directed, was dealt with more as a child than an adult, and was assumed to need the guidance of the parents and school to the extent that such could be provided. Many new college students are not prepared for the freedom college life offers. Many are on their own for the first time and are not sure what to do with such a degree of personal freedom. It is not unusual for the new college student to have more fun exploring the newly found freedom than exploring his or her studies. It takes time to find the balance between freedom and expectations.

A special case of this adjustment is reserved for the person who went to a small high school in which he or she was the class president, head cheerleader, football star, or debate champion. This person walks into college expecting the same adulation that was accorded in high school only to find that he or she is no longer recognized. Of course, the same could apply for a student from a larger school.

Essentially, the new college student is expected to assume the role of mature, independent adult with all the responsibilities it entails. The behavior that was encouraged or tolerated in high school will be seen as immature among college peers.

PROBLEMS OF THE HEAD-INJURED COLLEGE STUDENT

Beyond the problems most college students face, the head-injured college student faces numerous additional concerns related to the injury. A particular student may show all or only a few of the problems presented here. Understanding the individual student requires a careful assessment to see which problems apply and which do not.

The problems described in this section of the book are based on knowledge of brain functions and impairments coupled with knowledge of what is expected in college. As has been noted several times in this book, the research is lacking to be able to say how common these problems are and who is most likely among the head-injured students to have them. Until the research is conducted and presented, the problems described here may be considered highly probable.

Slow Mental Processing. Mental processing refers to the speed with which information coming into the brain or already in the brain is analyzed, organized and translated into an appropriate response. An example would be asking someone a question. How quickly was it comprehended? How long did it take for the person to respond? Was the response such that it indicated a real grasp of the question? Was the response realistic?

It is not unusual for the head-injured student to be slower in mental processing than he or she was before the injury, and slower than other students. Try to imagine the brain operating at a slightly slower speed than it should. The information is slower getting into the brain and being sent to other brain areas. Analysis of the information takes longer than it would for other people (just as early computers took longer to process information than present computers). The response may be slower in being formed and expressed. This slower mental processing makes it difficult for the head-injured student to take in information at the usually rapid pace one finds in college. If a number of information sources are being provided, such as a multi-media presentation with quickly changing scenes and varied musical backgrounds, the head-injured student will have even greater difficulty because so much has to be processed at the same time. A lecture or demonstration that quickly shifts from one area to another is more difficult than for other students. By the time the present material is processed, the lecture or demonstration is a step or two ahead of the student. The same applies to a group discussion in which many points are raised and many people are talking, often at the same time. This is difficult enough for the person without a head injury, but is especially so for the head-injured student.

Memory Impairment. Memory impairment is one of the most common indications of brain injury and remains one of the most common aftereffects. The type of memory impairment depends, of course, on the area of brain injury. As was noted previously, damage to the hippocampal areas in the temporal lobes will result in impairment of storing new information. Presumably (because we lack complete data), damage to the lobes of the brain will result in memory problems related to the functions of those lobes (for example, motor patterns in the frontal lobes or musical scores in the right hemisphere).

Impaired memory may be specific, such as for words, spatial locations, or emotional situations, but in most cases it is more general than specific. More often than not, the impairment will involve verbal and episodic events (recalling what was said and what has happened). In general, it is recent memory that is impaired in most cases (events within the past few minutes to hours). Long-term memory is usually left intact, such as memories of childhood events.

A necessary issue must be addressed here: whether memory itself is impaired or some other related function is actually responsible for what appears to be a memory problem. For example, it is possible that memory itself is intact, and the problem rests in the person's inability to keep attention on an event. It is obvious that if something is not noticed it will not be remembered. If someone talks to me and I am not paying attention because my mind is elsewhere, only part, or none, of what was said will be registered in my brain. Later, when I am asked to repeat what was said and cannot do so, a memory problem is assumed when actually it was an attentional problem. If the information had been registered, memory would have been quite adequate.

It is most important for the head-injured student to be properly tested to see just what part of the memory system is not functioning. To help the student we must have accurate knowledge of the impairment in order that it may be effectively addressed. This is most important, as it is quite likely that some degree of memory problem will be present in almost every head-injured college student.

Comprehension. Comprehension is essentially synonymous with understanding. A person's level of comprehension depends on mental alertness, intelligence and past experience. We would hardly expect a very young child who is mentally slowed by medication to understand (comprehend) the subtleties of diplomatic wording. While this is an admittedly extreme example, the same reasoning applies at other levels. We cannot expect a student with impaired abstract thought to understand some esoteric point of theory or the impact of numerous historical events as they relate to some present political point.

Because of slower mental processing and disturbances of verbal ability, many head-injured college students will experience some degree of difficulty in comprehension. Compared to their classmates, the head-injured student will have greater difficulty understanding demonstrations, lectures, or other educational experiences. This is not due to an impairment of overall intelligence; the person may be intellectually quite bright. Fellow students, professors, friends or family are likely to not understand why the student must be told several times how to do something or why the student must ask for clarification of the points that everyone else has already gotten. The head-injured student may begin to feel embarrassed by this impairment of comprehension that makes him or her appear mentally dulled when, in fact, he or she is intellectually quite adequate for the task.

The problem of comprehension is worse when the understanding rests on subtle points rather than clear, concrete ones. It is easier, for example, to understand a line from Shakespeare when it contains a precise point rather than a metaphor. Sometimes the problems in comprehension can hinge on the way something is worded or how it is combined with other material. A student may easily respond to, "Put the chemical in the container," but be unable to comply with, "Put the chemical in the container after writing the symbol." The simple word *after* changed the whole picture because it calls on a number of mental abilities that were not needed with the first request.

It is understandable that the uninformed observer is confused by the inability of the student to carry out a simple request (simple to the observer, I must add) or to understand a certain point that does not seem all that difficult. Although the student is acutely aware of the problem, it is often not clear to him or her *why* it is a problem. Generally, the student would have great difficulty giving an explanation to someone else as to why these seemingly "simple" tasks have become so hard.

Verbal and Written Expression. Although the correlation is not perfect, often when a person has difficulty with spoken expression, writing is also affected. For most people, these problems are related to impairments in the left hemisphere. The impairment may range from a full aphasic syndrome in which communication is seriously affected to lesser degrees of difficulty such as coming up with the name of something or someone (called anomia).

If the person is aphasic, comprehension of what is heard may or may not be preserved. In some forms of aphasia (e.g., Wernicke's or global aphasia) comprehension of spoken words is so impaired as to rule out college. In other forms of aphasia (e.g., Broca's aphasia) comprehension remains intact but the ability to express one's self is impaired. A person with a nonexpressive aphasia may be able to attend college if a way of expression can be found (e.g., the use of word boards in which the person points to or manipulates words on a magnetic board).

More prevalent than the full-blown aphasic syndromes are problems of speech and writing related to slow mental processing. The student is slower in understanding what has been said, and is slower in responding. He or she may be unable to find the right word, or words may be substituted for others. Speech may be slurred or scanning (slow, methodical speech), or there may be difficulties in pronounciation due to impaired muscle function (technically called dysarthia). In many cases, the person is aware of the speech or writing problem, but the awareness does nothing to alleviate them. It is common, in the early days of recovery, for the head-injured person to become depressed and frustrated that speech does not work as it should. Imagine the frustration of knowing what you want to say, but when it comes out the words are all wrong and you know it!

Greater Distractibility. It is known from work with public school children that distractibility is a common problem after head injury. The distractible student is less able to keep attention focused, as he or she should, on necessary aspects of the environment such as lectures or films being presented. Extraneous events call the person's attention away from important matters. For example, while a non-injured student is listening to a lecture the late entrance of another student may be ignored, unnoticed, or occasion for a quick glance. The head-injured student is likely to be more distracted by the late entrance and to lose his or her train of thought. The same would apply to any other extraneous source of distraction (e.g., a noise in the hall, student talking in another part of the room).

Distractibility becomes evident when the student is in a situation with many sources of information coming in at the same time, such as a professor lecturing while a slide show is being presented. If one cannot keep attention focused properly, which may require great effort, confusion is the result. As you sit reading this page you must keep your eyes in proper position, certain muscle groups must be functioning adequately, you must concentrate your attention on the words, and you must ignore a great deal that is going on around you. How well would you understand this page if you stopped to notice the color of the walls, a picture, a noise from the next room, every automobile that passed in front of the house, and two people talking softly? Fortunately, your brain has learned to filter out unnecessary stimulation so attention can be focused where it is needed. With head injury, this ability to focus attention is less well tuned.

Difficulty in Abstraction. The ability to think abstractly means the ability to think about something or respond to a situation beyond the concrete, literal event before us. If shown a red box, red flower, and red ball, and asked to tell what is the same about them you would immediately say they are all red. This requires abstract thought. The person with impaired abstraction, the person who thinks concretely, might reply there are no similarities across the three objects, or might give a concrete response such as all the items could fit into a box. Words are often used abstractly (actually, words are themselves abstract symbols because they stand for something else). To use words abstractly means to use them to convey something other than what the words literally mean. Expressions such as, "I'm on top of the world," to convey happiness, or, "My heart is broken," to convey sadness do not mean literally that a person is on top of the world or his or her heart is broken. Imagine taking these literally. A great deal of human communication uses such expressions with the assumption that the listener understands the abstract nature of the words.

Just as so many other impairments are variable, so is abstraction. It ranges from reasonably adequate to very seriously impaired. In varying degrees, difficulty in abstraction will lead the head-injured college student to miss points of history made by the professor, to have great difficulty understanding points of a theoretical nature, or to misunderstand the meaning of a poem or story that is rich in metaphors and similes. Much humor is based on abstraction, and the student may miss a humorous remark by the professor or another student. The head-injured student may then feel confused by the laughter of the other students. With abstraction difficulties, a student could easily conduct an experiment based on a step by step procedure, but fail an examination because he or she cannot see the similarities across various experiments.

Lower Stress Tolerance. The effects of brain injury and the stresses they produce as the person deals with everyday life combine to produce lowered stress tolerance. The lowered tolerance is in part physically based, but it is heightened by the person's recognition that he or she is not the same as before, and is having a harder time than other students. Irrespective of the underlying factors, it takes less stress for the head-injured student to become discouraged, depressed, frustrated, anxious, or irritable. The stresses another student may consider of no serious consequence may seem overwhelming to the head-injured student.

Lowered stress tolerance means the person is facing more stress than others because so many events are seen stressful. It is this personal perception of stress that determines how a person will physically and emotionally react, irrespective of how anyone else sees the situation. What is stressful to a person depends on his or her own definition. Of course, there may be no objective basis for the sense of threat the person feels, but the fear and stress are no less real to that person. For example, if a student has a strong fear of speaking in front of the class, being forced to do so will create very real stress, just as real as if the student were in physical danger.

Since the head-injured student may have lower stress tolerance, the result is more frequent stress-related complaints. He or she will be under more emotional tension and will more frequently have physical problems such as tension headaches, fatigue, or digestive difficulties. None of these reactions is helpful to a student who is already having some degree of difficulty with school.

Planning and Organization. As was noted previously, many people, including health and mental health professionals, do not understand that social judgment and awareness, and the abilities to plan, organize, schedule, and follow through with actions are brain fucntions. Most people are quick to understand that paralysis resulted from brain injury, but social and personality functions are relegated to the "psychological" domain. It must be recalled that the social and personality functions are mainly controlled by the prefrontal region of the frontal lobes, and that this region of the brain is very likely to suffer injury in most forms of accidents. The social and personality abilities may be impaired even in the absence of any physical disabilities that would indicate brain injury.

To get through college requires a great deal of planning and organization. The student must decide when to graduate and how to set up a semester by semester schedule to achieve that goal. How many hours, and what specific courses must be taken each time? Within the courses, assignments must be planned for completion at the correct time, and the demands of all courses must be organized into some pattern that can be dealt with effectively. Daily activities must be planned to insure meeting obligations and to avoid conflicts. Once the plans and patterns are established, the person must follow through with them.

Other people are often less than tolerant when the head-injured student fails to plan or organize, or fails to follow through with those plans if they are made. The other person may be dismayed by a schedule of classes that do not seem to meet any of the expectations for graduation. Again, being repetitious, such problems can result from brain injury and must be dealt with as such.

Given the prevalence of closed head injuries, including minor ones, and the high likelihood that the frontal and temporal lobes will be injured to some degree in many cases, the incidence of students with such difficulties is very likely high. College personnel must be alert to this possibility.

Emotions. Emotional reactions such as depression, anxiety, irritability or frustration are likely from both the physical aspect of the injury (e.g. damage in the limbic system or frontal-limbic connections) and the more psychological aspect of recognizing and coping with newly acquired impairments (i.e. stress). In other words, it is not possible to separate the physical from the psychological in understanding emotional reactions. There will be emotional reactions, with depression being the most common. Even if a clear physical basis for an emotional reaction cannot be established, the college student with a head injury is nonetheless facing great stresses as he or she perhaps realizes for the first time the true nature of the impairments (as cognitive abilities are now being put to the test). If there are physical difficulties as well, the person may now realize the extreme difficulty of getting around on a tight schedule. It is little wonder that the head-injured student feels a bit overwhelmed by it all (just as his or her non-injured fellow student may be feeling).

The sense of being overwhelmed, frightened, or simply unsure help generate the emotional reactions of the student. The non-injured student is likely to face many of the same emotional reactions, but without the additional knowledge that one has some brain-related problems.

Self Concept. As any person who has worked in rehabilitation knows, physical (or emotional) disabilities commonly create difficulties in the patient's self concept. Since most head-injured persons are aware to some degree of their problems, their self concept is likely to be altered. The person begins to feel less worthy because he or she cannot function physically or mentally as well as classmates. Unfortunately, the reactions of other people to the injured person often do not help. These reactions are often such that they reinforce the idea that the injured person is different in a negative way. As the student begins to acknowledge to himself or herself that there are limitations and that he or she will not be the same person, self concept begins to decline.

On a day to day basis, lowered self concept means the person is likely to be self-conscious and sensitive to criticism or rejection to the point that misunderstandings and misinterpretations occur. Confidence is lowered and the person gives up easily. The extreme of this problem would be a person who thinks so little of his or her abilities that college is not even attempted. In this situation, if college is attempted the person insures failure by not trying hard enough. While the lack of effort insures failure, the person views the failure as proof of the lack of abilities.

Perhaps, after a few success experiences, the self doubts will lessen and confidence will rise. Until they do, the student will continue to deal with a layer of psychological concerns that distract from the energy it takes to get through college.

Social Skills. The control of social skills rests primarily in the prefrontal region of the frontal lobes. If there is frontal lobe injury the person will very likely exhibit some degree of difficulty in social situations. The person is likely to be impulsive and may exhibit less good judgment than was shown pre-injury. He or she may speak in class when it is not appropriate, or may offer a suggestion in a meeting that is inappropriate or at least was not really wanted. A remark by the student about the physical appearance of another student may be seen as unnecessarily blunt. The student may join a group without being invited to do so. He or she may miss subtle clues or messages, and persist in a behavior until the other person reacts more forcefully. For example, the student may miss gentle, polite reminders that a classmate is engaged, eventually resulting in an unpleasant confrontation. The ability to benefit from the feedback of other people may be impaired to the point that the student seems to be not listening or to be unconcerned.

The very sensitive person is likely to be acutely aware of physical problems resulting from a head injury. He or she may spill a drink or bump into another person because of impaired motor coordination. The student then begins to avoid situations where such events might occur. Unfortunately, the student will very likely find invitations dwindling as others become uncomfortable or fearful the student might create a problem. The end result is the head-injured person becoming socially isolated and withdrawn, with some quite understandable emotional reactions as well.

Alcohol and Other Drugs. Given the widespread use of alcohol and other drugs on college campuses, this must be addressed as a special problem for the head-injured student. There are a number of factors that make the head-injured student a prime target for the use of these substances. He or she is facing a great deal of stress from the injury and from college, social judgment and control may be lowered, and there is a great deal of peer pressure to use the substances (beer busts, for example). As much as anyone, the head-injured student wants to fit in and feel a part of the total campus life. Unfortunately, head injury affects one's tolerance for many chemical substances, including alcohol. A dosage of alcohol or marijuana that at one time would have had minimal effect, may now create serious problems of judgment and control. If the person has a seizure disorder, from whatever cause, drugs, especially alcohol, lower the threshold for seizures. The interaction between alcohol and other drugs and the prescription medications the student may be taking may produce serious, potentially fatal effects. The concern over alcohol and other drugs is warranted when it is recalled that the most frequently head-injured person is a young male who was hurt in an alcohol-related automobile accident. Already having had a history of using alcohol or other drugs, the head-injured student is likely to hope to continue using them; thus, setting the stage for the problems described here.

Medications. It is standard procedure after major brain surgery or a serious head injury to prescribe anticonvulsant medication to prevent seizures, even if the person has not shown signs of such a disorder. Depending on a number of factors, anywhere from three percent to as high as 60 percent of head-injured individuals will ultimately develop seizures, but the problem may not become evident for several months or longer post-injury (Jennett, 1983b). It is certainly prudent to prescribe preventative doses of anticonvulsants. Of course, a person could be taking anticonvulsant medication for non-injury related seizures. In addition to anticonvulsants, the head-injured student may be taking medications for other injuries incurred at the time of the head injury. For example, he or she may be taking muscle relaxants, blood-thinning agents, and medications for orthopedic problems. Many of these medications can produce significant side-effects that interfere with college performance. Two of the more common side-effects are drowsiness and fatigue, but just about anything else is possible, ranging from dulling of mental abilities to headaches to tremors.

By the time the student with a head injury has added one medicine to another and another, the academic side-effects may be serious. If the student is using alcohol or other drugs in addition to the prescription medications, the effects are even worse. The student must discuss these potential problems with the prescribing physician or another physician who is intimately familiar with the drugs and how they interact with other drugs, especially in a head-injured person.

Fatigue. Fatigue in a brain-injured person comes from two sources. First, but not necessarily true for all cases, there may be physical problems of coordination and ambulation. If there are physical problems, everyday activities such as walking, picking something up, or turning a page in a book may become strenuous exercise for the person. The physical activities that many people take for granted as effortless become difficult and tiring for the injured person. By the time a full day has passed, the head-injured student has exerted a great deal more physical effort than his or her non-injured classmate.

Fatigue also comes from the mental strain it takes to concentrate, comprehend, or think. We do not often stop to realize that mental activity can be quite exhausting, but it is not hard to demonstrate. Just remember the last time you sat in a comfortable chair while a distraught friend, near emotional collapse, called on you to listen and help with a problem. In a very short time, you were exhausted. Remember the last time you spent all afternoon studying for an important examination. You exerted minimal physical effort, but your fatigue was very real. The use of mental energy can be exhausting. When all is said and done, mental activity is brain activity, and the brain is a working organ that uses a great deal of the body's energy. The brain is burning energy, and that energy is coming from the rest of your body; hence, the fatigue.

Because the head-injured person must often exert extra effort to keep his or her attention focused and to analyze incoming material, more energy is expended than for the non-injured person. By the time the physical and mental fatigue have combined, the student may simply want nothing more than to sit quietly for awhile. Even going to a concert, which you might consider relaxing, may be too much for the student who has already put in a full day of extra mental and physical effort. To the casual observer the head-injured student may appear apathetic or withdrawn, neither of which is true. If one has only so much energy, it must be expended wisely, and must be replenished regularly.

Unrealistic Expectations. It is the sincere hope of all those who incur an injury, and all those who care about that person, that he or she will return to pre-injury levels of function. It is a difficult burden to realize that hopes and dreams will not be realized, at least as they were originally envisioned. This alteration of plans sometimes leads the person, family, and friends to expect more from the patient than can realistically be produced. This is an attempt to deny the limitations by showing that one is as normal as ever. These expectations are sometimes directly expressed or they may be more subtly conveyed (but just as real).

In an effect to prove that everything is just as it was before the injury, the student may take a full academic load, work, and carry on a full social life. A college major may be selected more for its appearance value (to prove "normality") than its realistic potential. The end result is, if not failure, increased stress and perhaps lowered performance on the student's part.

In some cases, the unrealistic expectations result from the person genuinely not knowing he or she is brain injured, such as in a minor head injury. This person, or those around him or her, does not realize there are any limitations to be dealt with. Nonetheless, the effects are the same: the person sets expectations that are unrealistic. Unfortunately in this case, the student does not even know why school has become so difficult.

Lack of Understanding From Others. Generally speaking, the average person does not have a great deal of knowledge about brain functioning. Many professionals, including those likely to be working with college students (professors, counselors, or psychologists, for example), have limited knowledge of brain functioning and the effects of injuries. That these people do not have a detailed knowledge of brain functions is not a criticism, for they have no reason to possess such detailed knowledge. There are specialty areas such as neurology, neuropsychology, or brain-injury rehabilitation where there are professionals who do have the detailed knowledge and who would be quite willing to share it with others when it is needed.

Specifically within the college setting, since that is the focus of this book, the student is likely to face a wall of misunderstanding from those around him or her. If the student has a noticeable physical sign of the head injury, there may be a greater tendency to assume that cognitive problems are also brain related. However, in many cases with obvious physical indications of injury, other people are still not likely to view the cognitive impairments as related to the injury.

The misunderstanding is significantly worsened if the head-injured student does not have clear physical impairments. He or she walks perfectly, speaks clearly, seems alert and aware, has good coordination and has no scars at all. It seems incomprehensible to many people that their child's, friend's, or student's poor planning, fatigue, social inappropriateness, or slow processing could be a brain problem. This not only adds to the student's frustration, it potentially leads to misdirection in terms of advising. The head-injured students may be referred for counseling for "mental problems" that in fact are brain problems. The assumption that one is suffering psychological problems carries with it the assumption that discussing the problems will help alleviate them. This is clearly a false assumption in the case of a head-injured student. While counseling may be quite beneficial to the head-injured student, it is helpful to the extent that the brain injury is taken into account.

If a person has incurred an undiagnosed head injury the chances of misunderstanding are even worse. This is especially true of the head-injured person who does not start school for a long time after the injury. During the time between the injury and starting college the person may have impairments of cognition that go unnoticed because the abilities are not being used. For example, during several years of working in a repetitive, non-reading type of work, the person may do well. When he or she starts college, and new cognitive demands are encountered, the person may find memory less than expected, or new learning to be more difficult than originally thought.

Specific Brain Impairments. In addition to the general problems described thus far, it is important to note that the student will have those impairments related to the area of injury (or, in the case of diffuse injury, areas of injury). These specific impairments must be added to the more general ones the student may face. For example, the student who insists on going into engineering in spite of significant impairment of spatial abilities is going to have more problems than a student who acknowledges a problem and works around it.

OVERVIEW

I cannot leave this chapter without a reminder that the points brought out here may or may not apply in a specific case. Each person is unique and may or may not have the same kinds of difficulties as an apparently similar person. Not every head-injured student is going to have verbal impairments or altered social skills. It is the task of those who are working with the student to determine which of the problems are applicable and which are not. The categorical assumption that because a person is head-injured, he or she will have some specific impairment could well lead to intervention where none was needed.

CHAPTER 5

IMPROVING THE HEAD-INJURED STUDENT'S COLLEGE EXPERIENCE

ALTHOUGH the head-injured student will encounter a number of problems in college that others may not face, there are many ways of improving the chances of having a successful college experience. To help insure success, the student must be assessed for areas of impairments and strengths, and a program must be designed with those qualities in mind.

The best overall suggestion of a general nature for the head-injured college student or the person contemplating college is to proceed slowly at first. Caution is necessary in the early stages of this endeavor. There must be a period of time in which the head-injured person tests various abilities and finds out what will and will not be problem areas. Trying to start with a full academic load and a full social life does not allow an adequate assessment of skills. If the student takes on too many activities and problems begin to emerge, it is very difficult to filter out exactly what is creating those problems. If problem areas are not clear, addressing them becomes difficult, if not impossible.

It is preferable for the head-injured person to take a longer period of time to finish college than to become so overwhelmed at first that he or she withdraws from school. If the withdrawal was for legitimate reasons, by which I mean unavoidable reasons, then the person has made a wise choice and can go on to seek other important pathways to a satisfying life. If the withdrawal resulted from preventable causes, it is unfortunate that the person gave up a once important goal that was in fact obtainable. It is unnecessarily stressful that the person concluded college was out of the question when, in fact, the motivation and ability were there, but he or she became involved in an overwhelming situation that could have been avoided.

I cannot profess that the following list of suggestions is complete and that someone will not present a unique idea that is not contained here. Be that as it may, the following are suggestions that should help the head-injured student remain in college. Some of the suggestions will be appropriate for some students and not for others. A careful assessment will allow the best utilization of these suggestions.

ADVISING THE HEAD-INJURED COLLEGE STUDENT

The following suggestions are not in any order of importance, other than the first one. Because the research is lacking, there is no way to present these in the order of importance or frequency of need. Each suggestion must be considered for each student. It is important that we assume nothing, but should consider the applicability of each point, even if our initial impression is that the student will function well in that aspect of college.

Complete Neuropsychological Evaluation. A complete evaluation is the cornerstone of effectively advising the head-injured college student. Thorough physical and neuropsychological evaluations are a necessity in helping the person plan a college career. Since this section is concerned with the neuropsychological evaluation, I will not address the physical assessment other than to note that it must be done.

I cannot overemphasize the importance of the neuropsychological evaluation being conducted by a person (or persons) specifically trained in such assessments. The evaluation of neuropsychological abilities, that is, the behavioral and cognitive aspects of brain injury, requires specialized testing by a person trained in understanding brain functions and injuries. A professional who is not specifically trained in brain functions is not appropriate for this type of evaluation, regardless of any other credentials he or she may possess. Anyone can learn to give tests and score them, but correctly interpreting the results demands specialized training and experience. Unfortunately, there is no convenient checklist that can be used to decide if a person is or is not qualified to do a neuropsychological evaluation. Two general guidelines may be helpful. First, ask the professional about his or her training and experience in conducting such evaluations. The person must have had supervised training in the area. Second, ask for a referral from a person in one of the head-injury professions or contact a rehabilitation facility, medical school or university to obtain names of possible evaluators.

Many professionals contribute to the overall evaluation of the head-injured person. Besides neuropsychologists, there are physicians, nurses, occupational therapists, speech therapists, physical therapists, counselors, social workers, and aides just to name a few. Of course, the input from family, friends, teachers, or employers is needed for a complete understanding of the person. For the rest of this section I will focus on my area, neuropsychology, while acknowledging the equally important contributions of other professionals.

While there are two major batteries (groups of tests) for neuropsychological assessment, any given assessment may or may not include all the tests that make up those batteries. In some cases, tests are not given because there is clearly no reason to do so, or they simply cannot be administered because of the head-injured person's condition. In other cases, in fact, most cases, additional tests are given because some ability not addressed in the main batteries needs to be assessed. In other words, there is no precisely set battery of tests that must be given to every person tested. The testing is individualized to the person, giving whatever is necessary to fully understand the head-injured individual. Regardless of the specific tests given, a completed neuropsychological evaluation provides information on the person's cognitive (intellectual) functioning, psychological functioning, social skills, and to some degree, physical functioning. Many specific functions are tested, for example, attention, memory, comprehension, expressive ability, coordination, emotional condition, level of awareness of impairments, and tolerance level just to mention a few. For a more detailed discussion of neuropsychological testing see Golden (1981) or Lezak (1983), among many good sources.

For the head-injured person contemplating college, more is needed than a standard neuropsychological evaluation. Testing is needed in the academic and vocational areas as well. Achievement testing is needed to indicate how much a person has already accomplished in a given area such as reading, arithmetic, history or chemistry. Aptitude testing is needed to suggest the person's potential for learning in a specific subject. Beyond the academic area, testing is needed in vocational interests and skills to assess the person's potential for employment in a vocational setting. The neuropsychologist may or may not be skilled in the administration and interpretation of these academic and vocational tests. If not, an appropriate referral can be made for the testing.

Although there is no precise definition of when an evaluation becomes dated, it is important to have current information on the head-injured person. The longer it has been since the injury, the more likely the data are to be stable over time; but for the first year or two post-injury, there may be dramatic improvements in functioning. These improvements need to be documented and taken into account in advising the person about college. On the conservative side, I suggest that within the first two years post-injury any evaluation that is three or four months old is outdated.

College personnel who are working with the head-injured student need to obtain permission from the student to get copies of any evaluation reports that are pertinent to advising. If the reports are not understandable because of terminology or technical details, a nontechnical report should be requested. In the least, if there are any questions about the report, the writer should be contacted to offer clarification. Once the reports are obtained and understood the data may be used to effectively advise the student.

It may have occurred to the reader, "Why not ask the head-injured person about the effects?" The answer is that the person may not be aware of all the problems that could impact on college life. The head-injured person will frequently have some degree of memory impairment; thus, recall of all necessary points is unlikely. Obtaining reports is a way of being sure all important information is available.

Head-Injury Services. The prospective student should contact the colleges he or she hopes to attend to see if special services are offered for head-injured individuals. Virtually all colleges have services for disabled students, but this is not enough. Someone on the staff must be able to work specifically with head-injured students. As I have noted several times, working with brain-injured persons, especially those without any obvious physical symptoms or signs, takes specialized understanding of the problems the students may face.

While some colleges do offer specialized services for their head-injured students, the programs are not widely known (it took many letters and calls for me to find some of them). The college may not be convenient for the student, even if it does have special services. The fact that a college does not advertise specialized services for head-injured students does not mean it cannot or does not offer helpful services. Contact the college to find out what is available. In almost all cases, the programs dealing with disabled students are located in an office specifically for that purpose, or they are in the college counseling center.

If the college being considered does not offer head-injury services, before giving up hope of attending there it must be noted that it is possible to find a head-injury professional who will serve as an ancillary advisor to the student. This professional could help plan courses and programs and be available for counseling when needed. This is my second choice, simply because a person working in the college setting on a daily basis has a better idea of the differences between classes, professors, programs, and requirements. Also, the college worker will have a better idea of where to turn for specialized services on campus. Nonetheless, to maximize the potential for success, it is best to have informed help than to try it alone.

Campus Size. Because the head-injured person may well have some degree of physical impairment along with spatial difficulties or other cognitive impairments, it is generally advisable to seek a compact, well-organized campus. Junior or community colleges often offer such an arrangement, as do smaller four-year institutions. The larger and less well organized a campus, the greater the potential for problems in getting from one building to another in the amount of time allowed between classes. There is also a greater potential for confusion if spatial problems exist. If the new student finds there are no difficulties in getting around, physically and spatially, moving to a larger campus is always possible the next semester or year.

Beyond the sheer size of the campus, the larger a college is the larger the number of students to add to the general sense of confusion and disarray during class change time. More students mean larger classes, which means a greater potential for the head-injured student to become distracted or confused.

Overall, it is generally best to begin the college career at a smaller campus, many of which have excellent reputations. One does not have to go to a large institution to obtain a high-quality education and subsequent employment.

If the head-injured student has serious physical impairments, he or she must be sure the campus is easily accessible. While there are federal laws that mandate accessibility, there is wide latitude in how this is provided. Obviously, a college campus cannot be made smaller, and elevators cannot always be guaranteed to work as they should.

Auditing. Auditing a class means taking it for no credit. The auditor in the class may choose to complete assignments or to pass them by. Examinations may be taken or not taken, at the discretion of the student. Auditing a course is an excellent way to get a feel for college life and to test how difficult a particular subject may be. When auditing, there is a lack of pressure about how well one will do in a course. Unfortunately, this lack of pressure can work both ways. The lack of pressure can also lead to a carefree attitude since the course will not count anyway. If one does not take the course seriously, one cannot get a true assessment of performance and possible difficulties the student might face. If one chooses to audit a course, it must be taken as if he or she is a full time student in a class that will be counted toward graduation.

If the student is not yet ready to audit a course, there are other options. He or she could take a correspondence course or a local adult education course offered by the public school system. If a student has been out of school for awhile, it takes time to get back into the habit of studying and learning on a formal basis. While the adult education class is not the same as college, it is still an academic setting that requires studying and learning. In that sense, the adult education class is still valuable.

A correspondence course is dependent upon the person's ability to write effectively, as assignments are written and sent back to the instructor. This large amount of writing must be seriously considered before taking a correspondence course, especially if there are any problems in written expression, even minor ones. Also, correspondence courses are generally less structured than regular classes and are frequently self-paced. This self-paced approach is not realistic for most regular college courses. Given that planning and organization are not always at the optimum level, such an unstructured setting as the correspondence course may not be indicative of true college potential. If a correspondence course is attempted, someone should help the student maintain organization and scheduling.

Academic Load. The typical college student carries between 12 and 15 hours per semester. This means that he or she is actually in class that many hours per week. The number of credit hours for a specific course may range from 1 hour (it meets 1 hour per week) to 6 or more hours (that many hours per week), but most classes are for 2 or 3 hours. Thus a 15 hour credit load probably means the student has 5 different 3 hour courses. Since most colleges require around 120 hours to graduate, it is up to the student to fit this any way he or she pleases. Some students carry a lighter semester load and take longer to graduate, while others take a heavy academic load with the goal of graduating in less than the usual four years. A student with an 18 hour load could have as many as six 3 hour courses. Considering the amount of reading, studying, out of class work, and other requirements, it is obvious that 18 hours of college in a semester requires a great deal of time and clear mental abilities. Many students in their zeal to complete college as fast as possible hurt themselves in the long run by not doing as well academically as they could have with a lighter load. When it is time to apply for a master's or doctoral degree program the lower grades will hurt the chances of admission. Given the opportunity to apply for a job, it is not difficult to see that a student with a straight A grade point average will have the edge over a person with a C average, all other matters being equal.

Because of the difficulties the head-injured student faces, it is certainly advisable for him or her to take a light academic load for at least the first semester or academic year. By light load, I am referring to one or two courses. If these work out well, which may mean a grade of C if that is what the person is capable of, the academic load may be increased gradually. If judgment and impulsivity are presenting problems, the advisor, family, or friends must exert considerable pressure to keep the student from attempting a clearly unrealistic load.

The head-injured student may be quite capable of going to college if overloading does not occur. Granting that it may be frustrating to take an extra year or two to graduate, the consequences of trying to rush it are far worse. Even if the head-injured student does not directly experience academic problems, he or she is making the college experience unnecessarily stressful by trying to keep up with an unrealistic schedule.

Easier Courses. As a general rule, it is preferable to ease into a potentially stressful situation rather than to jump into it. It is generally better to build up to the stressful experience. If there are doubts about one's ability to go to college, it is best to start with classes that are familiar and relatively easy for the person. All people have areas of study that are easy for them, and other areas that are quite difficult. It makes little sense, given that the student has choices, to take the difficult, frustrating, stressful classes the first semester. It is better for the student to experience success and pleasure in the early days of college. At some point, the difficult courses must be confronted, but there is usually no rule that says they must be crammed into the first semester. Of course, certain courses may be required in the first semester or two, but this usually applies to only a few courses, if at all.

If the head-injured student has always been good in a certain subject such as English or chemistry, he or she should begin with those familiar subjects. If it occurs to the reader that the head-injured student is taking the evasive or easy way out, let me point out that all the courses are needed at some point, so why not take them when they serve the greatest purpose? The student is taking the sensible way, not the evasive way. It is just a matter of timing, and it is better for the student to begin with a good feeling about college and his or her chances of being successful.

In advising the student it is important that grades in high school or previous college classes be checked. A student's memory of enjoying a class may also be remembered as having done well in it, when, in fact, the grades were not that good. If there are memory problems, the accuracy of recall is not reliable. Whether or not a course will be easy for a student depends on the injuries he or she has incurred. A pre-injury class that was enjoyable and which resulted in a high grade may now be difficult and frustrating, especially so because of the past high performance.

Talk to the Professors. The image many people have of a college professor is usually far removed from the actual person. Among many students there is a rather generalized fear or dread of talking to the professor. The student is frequently afraid of interrupting some important matter, or perceives the professor as too busy to be seriously concerned about the student. Students often view the academic process as one in which rules cannot be altered, demands cannot be changed, or requirements cannot be shifted. In fact, the professor has tremendous flexibility in how to conduct a class and the types of requirements he or she wishes to impose on the class. Unfortunately, too many students have taken advantage of this flexibility and expected alterations that, if granted, would create chaos. Functioning in the real world requires that one learn to live within the rules, but, on occasion, exceptions can and should be made.

Most professors are more than willing to discuss the special needs of students with a legitimate reason to request an exception to the usual requirements. Examinations may be scheduled on an individual basis if the person needs a reader or more time is needed to complete the examination. The professor will not lower the standards for the course, and the serious student would not expect that anyway, but the professor may be quite willing to allow extra time for a paper, or to allow less class participation than is usually expected. If questions arise as to whether or not an exception is warranted, the college's disabilities services or the counseling center is usually able to verify the need. It is unfortunate that too many times professors have found out their flexibility has been abused, so do not be offended if there are some initial questions about why the exception is needed.

At the college level, not just in the classes themselves, if there are requirements such as writing examinations or other graduation requirements that are likely to create problems for the head-injured student, the student should contact the person in charge of the program to see if there are alternate ways to meet the requirement. It is unreasonable to expect a college to suspend requirements that are an integral part of the college degree; but with legitimate cause, alterations can be made to accommodate the special needs of the student. It is always best to ask rather than assume there is no way around an obstacle.

When approaching the professor or college administrator remember he or she is a person, and the image is probably very different from that real person. When talking to the person it is best to give a brief explanation of the problems and how they affect course or other academic requirements. Explain to the person as precisely as possible what is desired in terms of alterations. In other words, have a plan, not just a general expectation that some kind of exception should be made. For example, it would be better to ask for an extra hour on an examination than it would be to simply tell the professor examinations are problems and expect him or her to offer a solution.

If the professor feels exceptions cannot be made, there is little the student can do if the class requirements are reasonable and are not arbitrarily enforced. If exceptions are not possible, the student may take the course from another professor, if possible, or see if another course may be substituted for the first one. In most cases, it is quite likely that a legitimate request will be met with a favorable response from the professor or college administrator.

Special Services. Virtually all colleges have either special services or a person on the staff who can offer such services when needed. By special services I am referring to help with reading, writing, arithmetic, computers, or whatever might happen to be available. These services are commonly called laboratories, such as the math laboratory or reading laboratory. These labs are designed specifically to offer assistance to the student who is having trouble in a given subject, head-injured or not. In some cases the services are offered at scheduled times, while in other cases the student may come and go any time the lab is open. Most campuses also offer very brief courses or workshops that address common campus concerns such as theme writing or how to effectively take an examination. In whatever form they are offered, these laboratories offer specialized, personalized services for the student. As soon as the student comes to the campus, or preferably before that, he or she should ascertain which services are offered to see if those he or she needs are available.

Beyond the more formal laboratories, most classes offer special study sessions, or groups of students may form their own study groups. Such opportunities should be utilized.

Seeking special services can be a psychologically threatening affair. It is an admission that one needs help, and this can be embarrassing. The risk of embarrassment may be so great as to prevent the student from getting the help he or she needs. In response to this, I will point out that college is not a high school in which the student seeking help is likely to be made fun of or ridiculed. To the contrary, in the college setting the student is likely to be respected for acknowledging the problem and doing something about it. Most people, including the professors, will not know the student is in a special laboratory unless the student tells them, and even then it will be of no consequence one way or the other.

The need for special services is much greater than many people realize, and many bright students take advantage of them. It is far better to acknowledge the existence of a problem than to try to hide it and only worsen the chances of successfully completing college. Denying the problem will not make it go away. The services for help are there, they are almost always free, and they should be utilized.

Classroom Aids. Recall that slowness of mental processing and memory difficulties are common among head-injured students. These difficulties present very real impediments to keeping up with a class, especially in terms of note taking and following demonstrations.

Taking notes in class requires quick thinking and quick writing responses. There must be an immediate decision as to what to write down and what may be left unwritten. It is evident that if mental processing is slow or memory is impaired, note taking can become quite difficult. Poor notes can be worse than no notes if they mislead the student. Prior to examination time, a review of poorly taken notes can create not only misinformation but a sense of anxiety as the student realizes the notes are unclear, incorrect, or inadequate.

Tape recording lectures or videotaping demonstrations is an invaluable way to compensate for poor note taking. After class is over the student can immediately review the class material and if he or she chooses can write down notes (pacing the writing appropriately) or store the tapes for later review. The tapes may then be reviewed as often as is necessary to achieve adequate comprehension of the material. Even if the head-injured student chooses to take notes during class, a tape recording would be beneficial, at least initially, to allow verification of the notes. If other people in the class are also recording, an arrangement can be worked out to share the tapes and reduce the expenses involved. I recommend having personal tapes just to be sure they are available when needed. If a class must be missed, it is not difficult to get another student to record the material, or most professors would be quite willing to record the material if a recording machine, tapes, and instructions are provided.

Even with tape recording, it is advisable for the head-injured student to find a willing person (classmate, friend, family) who will attend the classes that are likely to present problems for the student. This is necessary to provide someone who can help clarify a point or help grasp an unclear demonstration. The head-injured student may need someone to help discuss a point, and it is most beneficial for that person to have heard exactly the same lecture or to have seen the demonstration. This is especially critical when something in the class did not get recorded, such as the comments of a student in another part of the room, or a visual display without sound.

Outside of class, if there are visual or physical impairments that prevent reading effectively, a reader should be obtained. Not only can this person read the material, but he or she is there to help clarify points and to discuss a topic while it is fresh in mind. The best place to start obtaining a reader is the college counseling center, which often maintains a list of such people.

Tutor. A tutor is a person who is knowledgeable in a subject and who offers individual instruction and help in that subject. The tutor and student work out mutual times for these sessions, ranging anywhere from daily to once a week or less. In some cases the tutor serves on an as-needed basis. Occasionally one will see a bulletin board notice offering tutorial services, but more often than not the potential tutor has not seriously thought about it but would be willing to do so if asked. Most colleges maintain a list of potential tutors, but if one is not available check with the counseling center, disabilities services, or the department office for that subject. Be prepared to pay the person for tutorial services.

Do not assume that just because a person is offering tutorial services he or she is necessarily good. Ask for references or permission to talk to a professor about the potential tutor. The receiving student must judge whether or not the services being provided are helpful, and must be ready to seek another tutor if necessary. Some students are very bright in their academic area, but they do not have the ability to convey that knowledge effectively or the patience to work with someone who is having trouble in an area that seems so easy for him or her.

Since a tutor may be brought in at any time, there is no reason to automatically assume one is needed. If it is already known that a particular subject is going to be difficult it is best to start with a tutor immediately. If the level of difficulty of a course is not predictable, there is no great harm in taking a short time to see how the course progresses. Never wait to obtain a tutor until the studies are so far behind that catching up is difficult or impossible.

Scheduling. As I have noted several times, there is a fairly high likelihood that the head-injured student will have some degree of difficulty in planning, organizing, and scheduling (because of the common occurrence of prefrontal injury). To help counter these problems it is important to begin a habit, perhaps already begun in the rehabilitation program, of writing down a schedule. Carrying a small notebook of schedules is a necessity for some head-injured students, and a helpful aid for others. Writing down names, dates and schedules is a necessity because memory is often impaired to some degree, and the notes help keep clear when an event occurs, where one should be, or which of two competing events should be attended.

A daily schedule should be filled in at the time an appointment is made or a time is set for an event or meeting. Waiting to write them down later may easily result in them not being written down at all (have we not all done this on occasion?). Just because a class meets at a regular time does not mean the person will remember it. Just because an appointment is set for the same time each week does not insure recalling it. All necessary information must be written down. Any cancellations can be readily scratched off.

On the same or a separate notebook, a schedule of more long-term commitments must be maintained. Once a due date is established for a paper, the head-injured student must not only write down the date, but he or she must also include specific times for getting the paper or other assignments done. Time must be scheduled for the library, the writing, the typing, and the reviewing. As much as possible, definite times should be noted, not general reminders. The note should say, "Study algebra from 10:00 AM to 11:00 AM," not, "Study today." Social events must be included in the schedule, as well as any other appointments the person may have.

The degree of scheduling required depends of course on the memory and planning ability of the student, but some scheduling is likely to be beneficial. Many non-injured students keep detailed schedules, as do most people with a busy life.

It is sometimes tedious and frustrating to have to write down everything, but failing to do so is worse. It takes only a few missed examinations or appointments to leave the impression that the student cannot be trusted to follow through with commitments. When this impression is conveyed to potential employers, the student may have difficulty getting hired, not because of the brain injury, but because of the problems in meeting necessary commitments. It would be unfortunate for a bright, capable student to be seen as irresponsible simply because he or she felt it was a burden to keep a written schedule. After many years of teaching, most college professors still take notes to class, even though they know the material well. They simply want to be sure that all necessary points have been covered. Most professors have calendars on which they write appointments. If the college professor, the busy homemaker, or the person in business needs to keep written schedules, there is no cause for embarrassment for the head-injured student to do the same.

Buddy System. It is important for the head-injured student to find a person who is willing to help him or her insure that all is going well. This person's role is to insure that the more or less technical details of everyday college life are met. He or she would help schedule the semester and how to meet class requirements, as well as social events or other appointments. The person may call the student to remind him or her of an appointment. It would be beneficial if the person attended the same classes as the head-injured student. This person would not necessarily have to be a student, but it would be helpful if he or she were one.

While such a system may appear to be an infringement on the independence of the head-injured student, it is certainly not. As I have noted previously, pretending something is not a problem does not make it go away. To establish such a system is to recognize there is a need and to address that need. If such assistance helps the head-injured student successfully complete college and go on to satisfying employment, it was obviously worth it.

Living Arrangements. If one asks two different head-injury specialists about where the head-injured college student should live, two different answers may be given. Both answers have their valid points, but the lack of research on the topic prevents any conclusive statements about the optimal type of living arrangement.

The first answer about where the head-injured student should live is that he or she should live anywhere he or she pleases, including group settings. Thus, if the person wants to live in a dormitory, fraternity or sorority house, or shared apartment or home, it should be promoted. The reasoning behind this approach is that the head-injured student needs to be as much a part of the regular college life as is possible. Also, living in some kind of group arrangement will help prevent the social isolation and sense of being different that are not healthy for the student. People will be available to offer whatever assistance is needed. The head-injured student will feel more like the typical college student.

The second answer is that the head-injured student should not try to live in a dormitory, fraternity or sorority house, or large group apartment or home. As anyone who has lived in such a setting can attest, such arrangements are often noisy, distracting, sometimes slightly chaotic, and hardly conducive to serious studying. Stereos are blaring, people are going up and down halls and talking back and forth, televisions are going, radios are on, and people are coming and going at various hours. I certainly do not want to leave the impression that such arrangements have no quiet time, for they do. However, consider a dormitory or other large arrangement. How well can one keep order with several hundred young, healthy, active college students?

I favor the second answer, that the head-injured student should avoid group living arrangements. The head-injured student is more likely than not to be easily distracted, to have trouble concentrating, to need more time than others to keep up with classes, and to be in greater need of rest because of the fatigue that is so common. These needs are not likely to be met in a group living situation, which not only means the denial of the needs, but added frustration for the student. I must point out that there is nothing "regular" or typical about living in a dormitory or other such arrangement. Many college students live on their own, at home with their parents, or in small shared apartments or houses. The college experience is no less because one did not live in some other setting.

The typical head-injured student would benefit from a quiet, orderly living arrangement. He or she may live at home, in a house or apartment alone or with a roommate or two who have been carefully selected, or in a college setting if a special quiet area has been set aside. These quiet arrangements will minimize distraction and will allow the head-injured student sufficient uninterrupted time to keep up with studies.

If the prospective student feels very strongly about living in a group setting such as a dormitory, two points should be considered. First, delay the group living arrangement for at least a semester to allow the student time to adjust to the other aspects of college life and to see what kinds of problems might arise in meeting the demands of his or her classes. Second, if the student still wants to live in the group setting, be sure a person is appointed to monitor the student's adjustment and grades. The outside monitor is needed because problems are not always apparent to the involved person when he or she is in the middle of a situation.

The main concern with a head-injured person living by himself or herself is that social isolation will set in. This may be true, but there is no reason it has to occur. There are a multitude of opportunities for social interaction on a college campus and the student must be encouraged to take advantage of them. This is a case where the buddy system would be most beneficial—someone who will be sure the head-injured student is aware of opportunities for social interaction. I must point out that living in a group setting does not insure social involvement.

Where the head-injured should live to maximize the chances of college success must be assessed in light of his or her unique status. Life choices are not always easy, and sometimes one factor must be traded off against another. If the head-injured student is prone to depression and isolation, a group setting might be preferable but the trade off will be in terms of academic performance and other stresses. The student and those working with him or her must discuss what is most important for the student, and find the best possible arrangement to accomplish that goal.

Counseling. It is important for the head-injured student to seek counseling whenever problems arise, irrespective of the nature of those problems. One of the frustrations mental health professionals face is that too many people allow problems to go on for a very long time before seeking help. By the time the person comes for help, the problems have mushroomed out of proportion, have become long-standing, and are much more difficult to alleviate than if the person had sought help when the problem first arose. This applies as much to the head-injured student as to the non-injured individual. Putting off counseling may well allow a small problem to become a large one.

Imagine a head-injured student who at the time of his or her first examination does not do well because of poor study habits (or any other reason). If the student seeks help immediately, new study habits can be discussed and other problems can be addressed (such as a sense of failure). If the student waits until the last of the semester to seek help, the grades in the course are probably so low that there is no way to redeem them. The student becomes discouraged, feels like a failure, and contemplates the possibility of not continuing in college. All of this could have been avoided if better study habits or other problems had been addressed earlier in the semester, allowing the opportunity to raise the course grade.

Imagine another student who is becoming depressed as he or she realizes the stresses of college life. If counseling is sought early in the semester, or whenever the problem arises, counseling or perhaps medication if necessary can be offered to help the student through the difficult times. If counseling is not sought, the depression worsens and small problems begin to look larger than they really are. Assignments remain uncompleted, classes are missed because the person does not feel like getting out. A downward spiral begins that ultimately creates an overwhelming situation for the student. The problem could have been significantly lessened by simply dropping a class, thereby reducing the stress level and sense of being overwhelmed. Perhaps a different living arrangement could have provided a better environment for studying. If the student waits too long to address the problems, an effective resolution may be difficult.

Virtually all colleges offer counseling services which are offered for no charge or a minimal fee. Of course, if the student has a trusted professional from past contacts, that person may be utilized if the student has any reservations about going to the college counseling center (a common fear is that other students will see him or her going for counseling). Even if the problem the student is facing is not directly related to the head injury, it is still desirable that the counselor or other professional have knowledge of head injuries.

It has been my experience with students and non-students with head injuries that a forthright, open discussion is almost always appreciated by the individual. In most cases the person is aware to some degree that something is not right, and there is a sense of relief to realize that cognitive or emotional problems are medically related, that is, related to the head injury. At first glance it may seem peculiar that a person would feel a sense of relief at such news (perhaps the word relief is a bit too strong, but the reaction is something close to it). Upon closer examination though, hearing that a symptom is related to the head injury relieves the person of the common fear that he or she is developing emotional or psychological problems. The head-injured person now has a better understanding of himself or herself, and some of the mystery is removed.

If the person chooses not to openly discuss the effects of the head injury, it is his or her right not to do so. A person cannot be forced to talk about anything. Efforts to force a discussion usually meet with direct resistance or with the person psychologically ignoring the counselor. Regardless of how well-meaning the intentions, the effort to force a person to confront a problem he or she is not ready to deal with usually fails. The person must decide when he or she is ready to open up about problems.

Support Groups. A support group simply means a group of people who share a common concern and who are willing to sit down with each other and discuss that concern and ways to deal with it. It may be lead by a professional or it may be a lay group, meaning the people themselves conduct the sessions. The support group can be an invaluable source of information, help, suggestions, and security. With or without professional leadership, support groups are often immensely beneficial. Support groups for head-injured persons are growing rapidly, many without professional leadership, yet quite effective.

On the college campus there are associations for most interest groups, including disabled students, and perhaps one specifically for head-injured students. If one is not available, the office of disabilities services or the counseling center are good places to start in forming one on campus. Of course, students do not have to formally establish anything. A group of students may wish to meet informally, rather than going through the formal procedure of establishing an officially recognized group.

Correlating Academic Areas With Abilities. Except for the occasional genius, no person can be good at everything, head-injured or not. Some students take history as if it were an old friend, while others just barely pass. Some students find psychology easy and enjoyable, while others who are equally bright, simply endure it. The head-injured student will not be equally capable in all subjects any more than the noninjured student. In addition, though, the head-injured student will have problems related to the injury, and these problems may make certain subjects even more difficult. For example, with right hemisphere injury, music or engineering may be precluded. With left parietal damage the student may be unable to pursue a mathematics major.

While common sense, combined with a knowledge of brain functions and dysfunctions, might suggest that certain academic subjects will be difficult with certain kinds of injuries, I cannot overemphasize the necessity of research to explore those common sense observations. Common sense does not always directly correlate with the reality of a situation.

It is the task of the student and those working with him or her to mesh the strengths and weaker areas with the requirements of a given academic subject. For the time being, this process is somewhat imprecise in that the empirical data are lacking that would allow the advisor to make more definitive statements. Future research will eventually allow the advisor to be more certain about which kinds of injuries present which kinds of difficulties in the college setting. In other words, the new data will help refine the process of advising the head-injured student. Until that time, advising must proceed on the basis of reasonable judgment.

SUMMARY

The suggestions brought out in this chapter must always be considered in light of the individual being advised. Not all head-injured students will have all the problems discussed in this book, and they will obviously not need intervention for all of them. As I have noted several times, we should assume nothing about the nature of functions and dysfunctions simply because the person is head-injured. He or she must be understood individually to allow the best utilization of our present knowledge.

CHAPTER 6

FUTURE DIRECTIONS

A GREAT DEAL remains to be done in the study of the head-injured college student, but the outlook appears active and hopeful. In closing this book, a number of issues related to future directions must be addressed: the improving rehabilitation possibilities, the need for controlled research, suggestions for the college system's manner of dealing with the head-injured student, and suggestions for where interested readers may turn for further information.

IMPROVING REHABILITATION POSSIBILITIES

As many authors have noted, for example, Begali (1987), the chances of recovering from a head injury are significantly greater today than they were just ten years ago. As medicine has improved its techniques for treating the head-injured individual, more and more people live. This means that more and more people will need head injury rehabilitation services. In the past ten years there has been a dramatic growth in the number of facilities designed specifically for head injury rehabilitation. The field of head injury rehabilitation is growing and learning as more and more people enter the rehabilitation process. This growth and learning will ultimately help produce innovative and sophisticated new ways of helping the head-injured person. For example, computers are now used in such programs as improving hand-eye coordination and memory retraining. As knowledge of brain injuries and rehabilitation increases, the techniques used today will be more finely tuned to the client's needs.

One can only imagine what new techniques will be introduced in the future that will have a dramatic impact on the lives of head-injured people.

The rapid growth of medicine in this area opens fascinating possibilities for dealing with the head-injured person: new imaging techniques such as magnetic resonance imaging, and microsurgery, just to name two. As medical techniques improve and the rehabilitation of the head-injured person becomes even more sophisticated, it is reasonable to assume that more and more people with head injuries will entertain the possibility of going to college.

FUTURE RESEARCH NEEDS

As I have stated many times in this book, there is a desperate need for controlled research on the head-injured college student. The first need refers to the rehabilitation process.

As Miller (1984) pointed out, many of the rehabilitation techniques used today have not been subjected to rigorous experimental investigation to test their effectiveness. In order to find the best techniques overall, and the best match between a person and a technique, research must be conducted to establish that improvement in a client is actually due to the techniques used. For example, we must establish that the improvements are not due to the passage of time and the natural healing of the brain that would have occurred anyway. Research will allow the rehabilitation expert to best judge what kinds of therapies should be used, and with whom.

We need basic data on the head-injured college student. At present, we have no information on the number of head-injured students. We have no data on how many head-injured students finish college and how many withdraw (and why they withdraw). Without continuing *ad infinitum* with possibilities, it is essentially correct to say that whatever question is asked about the head-injured college student, the answer will be based on experience, not research. The need for these basic data cannot be overstated. It is difficult to establish a program, which is often a very expensive enterprise, without information as to how many students will need it and utilize it.

The research on head-injured college students must address an issue I have raised several times in this book: the student who is unaware of an injury or its effects. These are the students who either do not know they have sustained an injury or who are unaware of the residual effects of a known injury (such as in a minor head injury). Personal experience tells me there are many more of these college students than one might expect, but research must be conducted. Personal experience is not enough.

Future research must address the issue of what kinds of impairments correlate with what kinds of problems in college. As I noted previously, while some of the correlations appear obvious, it takes controlled research to provide definitive answers. It would be unfortunate to advise a student away from a chosen area of study only to later find that there are exceptions and that he or she could have succeeded. It would be equally unfortunate to tell a student that a given academic subject will present no problems, only to find out that it involves some cognitive skill that was not apparent and which the person lacks. We need a careful analysis of the cognitive skills that are needed in the various academic areas. Superficial observation is not enough. We have to know what specific cognitive skills and personality traits are necessary for a specific subject. This research must be repeated many times (replicated), because researchers know that one study does not offer definitive proof about a subject. If many studies show the same results, the conclusions are more likely to be correct.

Another need for future research is to address the relationship between the head-injured college student's school performance and the actual workplace. We cannot automatically assume that what is seen in college will transfer to the job. This can work both ways. Sometimes the brilliant student is less than brilliant on the job, and the student who did less well in college turns out to be a brilliant worker. Specifically in reference to the head-injured student, a careful analysis must be made of the demands of various jobs in light of the capabilities of the head-injured person.

Future research must provide answers as to the frequency with which the problems described in Chapter 4 actually occur. Designing effective, efficient programs to help the head-injured students requires utilizing resources to their best advantage. It would make little sense to design a regular all-day workshop for a cognitive problem that only one or two students have. Their concerns could be better addressed in personal or group sessions.

Finally, the research must explore the best ways for different students to approach college. While common sense now dictates a slow and careful approach to beginning college, there is no *research* to show that such an approach is best for all students. It would be helpful to have a number of step by step programs for various kinds and levels of brain injuries. There cannot be a single best way for all head-injured students to start college or resume it. Perhaps for some people it would be better to start in a junior college, for others an adult education class might be preferable, yet others may begin in a four year college.

SUGGESTIONS FOR COLLEGES

A number of suggestions may be offered for colleges and their personnel. These may be implemented with a minimal amount of expense and effort.

Survey. Each college should do its own research now, rather than to wait for a national study. Even with a national study, the data remain just that: national. A particular college may have more or less head-injured students than the national average, and the types of problems may differ from the national data. The ideal way to obtain these data would be to ask all students at the time of enrollment (for example, on the enrollment form). If this is not possible, a large number of students could be contacted at random to obtain the necessary data, with the assumption that the sample reflects the college as a whole. Even then, some students will be missed because they are unaware of their injury or the effects of a known injury.

Head-Injury Services. On any particular college campus there may or may not be a special service for head-injured students. If a separate office is not justified, the campus should have a person on the staff who is specifically trained to work with head-injured students. However the college chooses to deal with the need, at least one person on the campus, preferably more than one person, must understand head injuries. This person can serve as a resource for other college personnel. In terms of training, this person must have had specific training and experience in a supervised setting. A one or two day workshop would be a good starting place, but is not enough training. A new person could be employed, or a present staff member could take a leave to receive training. If a leave is not possible, time for training could be included in the position.

College Staff Training. Available staff or outside consultants should be called upon to conduct seminars and other types of training about the head-injured student. The purpose of such training would not be to make the recipients (professors, residence hall advisors, counselors, and other college staff) experts, but to raise awareness of the problem. Awareness will result in better referrals and handling of students' needs.

Brain Injury Courses. College programs that train people to work with students in a nonrehabilitation setting must include coursework and experience in detecting brain injuries and working with the head-injured student. Programs such as psychology, counseling, and student personnel, to name some, need such courses. Although these programs are usually at the master's or doctoral level, the courses need not be restricted to graduate students.

RESOURCES

It is appropriate to close this book with some suggestions for resources where one might turn for information about head injury. As of this writing, I am not aware of any centralized clearing house about college programs specifically designed for the head-injured student.

The best single source for general information about head injuries is the National Head Injury Foundation, Inc. The current address of the NHIF is:

National Head Injury Foundation
333 Turnpike Road
Southborough, MA 01722

Virtually all states now have a state head injury association whose address may be obtained from the national organization or by asking any head-injury professional.

Among others, the United States Government has two agencies that are directly involved in information about head injuries. They are:

National Institute of Neurological and Communicative Disorders and Stroke
Department of Health and Human Services
Bethesda, MD 20014

and

Rehabilitation Services Administration
Department of Education
Washington, D.C. 20202

Two information centers were especially helpful in providing resources used for this book, and in referring me to other resources I was unaware of. They are:

National Rehabilitation Information Center
4407 Eighth Street, N.E.
Washington, D.C. 20017

and

Heath Resource Center
One Dupont Circle, Suite 800
Washington, D.C. 20036

Specifically in reference to whether or not a college has a head-injury program, as I noted earlier I am not aware of any central clearing house for such information. The best way to obtain the information is to contact the college in question. If the college has a staff member who belongs to the Association on Handicapped Student Services Programs in Postsecondary Education (AHSSPPE), he or she will have access to current information about the programs known to that organization.

BIBLIOGRAPHY

Adams, R.D., and Victor, M.: *Principles of Neurology,* 3rd ed. New York, McGraw-Hill, 1985.

Bauer, W.R., and Titonis, J.: Management and Advocacy. In Ylvisaker, M., and Gobble, E.M.R. (Eds.): *Community Reentry for Head Injured Adults.* Boston, College-Hill, 1987.

Begali, V.: *Head Injury in Children and Adolescents.* Brandon, VT, Clinical Psychology Publishing Company, 1987.

Bolger, J.P.: Educational and Vocational Deficits. In Rosenthal, M., Griffith, E., Bond, M., and Miller, J.: *Rehabilitation of the Head Injured Adult.* Philadelphia, F.A. Davis, 1983.

Caveness, W.F.: Incidence of craniocerebral trauma in the United States in 1976 with trends from 1970 to 1975. *Advances in Neurology, 22:* 1, 1979.

Cook, J. (Ed.): *The ABI Handbook Serving Students With Acquired Brain Injury in Higher Education.* Sacramento, California Community Colleges, 1987.

Cook, J., and Knight, N. (Speakers): *Assessing Students With Acquired Brain Injury in Higher Education.* (Cassette Recording.) San Diego, Convention Recorders, 1987.

Cook, J., Knight, N., and Harrington, D. (Speakers): *Serving Students With Acquired Brain Injuries in Higher Education.* (Cassette Recording.) San Diego, Convention Recorders, 1986.

Gardner, H.: *Frames of Mind.* New York, Basic Books, 1983.

Gluhbegovic, N., and Williams, T.H.: *The Human Brain: A Photographic Guide.* Hagerstown, Harper and Row, 1980.

Golden, C.J.: *Diagnosis and Rehabilitation in Clinical Neuropsychology,* 2nd ed. Springfield, IL, Charles C Thomas, 1981.

Golden, C.J., and Anderson, S.: *Learning Disabilities and Brain Dysfunction: An Introduction for Educators and Parents.* Springfield, IL, Charles C Thomas, 1979.

Hackler, E., and Tobis, J.S.: Reintegration into the Community. In Rosenthal, M., Griffith, E., Bond, M., and Miller, J.: *Rehabilitation of the Head Injured Adult,* Philadelphia, F.A. Davis, 1983.

Hall, D.E., and DePompei, R.: Implications for the head-injured reentering higher education. *Cognitive Rehabilitation, May/June:* 6, 1986.

Halstead, W.C.: *Brain and Intelligence.* Chicago, University of Chicago Press, 1947.

Hartlage, L.C., and Telzrow, C.F. (Eds.): *The Neuropsychology of Individual Differences.* New York, Plenum, 1985.

Hebb, D.O.: Intelligence in man after larger removals of cerebral tissue: report of four left frontal lobe cases. *Journal of General Psychology, 21:* 73, 1939.

Holmes, C.B. (Speaker): *The Head-Injured College Student.* (Cassette Recording.) Shawnee Mission, KS, Kansas Head Injury Association, 1987.

Holmes, C.B.: The head-injured college student: the rehabilitation perspective. Unpublished manuscript, 1988.

Jennett, B.: Scale and Scope of the Problem. In Rosenthal, M., Griffith, E., Bond, M., and Miller, J.: *Rehabilitation of the Head Injured Adult.* Philadelphia, F.A. Davis, 1983a.

Jennett, B.: Post-traumatic epilepsy. In Rosenthal, M., Griffith, E., Bond, M., and Miller, J.: *Rehabilitation of the Head Injured Adult.* Philadelphia, F.A. Davis, 1983b.

Kolb, I.Q., and Whishaw, B.: *Fundamentals of Human Neuropsychology,* 2nd Ed. New York, Freeman, 1985.

Levin, H.S., Benton, A.L., and Grossman, R.G.: *Neurobehavioral consequences of closed head injury.* New York, Oxford, 1982.

Lezak, M.D.: *Neuropsychological Assessment,* 2nd Ed. New York, Oxford, 1983.

Luria, A.R.: *Higher Cortical Functions in Man.* New York, Basic Books, 1966.

Luria, A.R.: *The Working Brain.* New York, Basic Books, 1973.

Marshall, L.F., and Marshall, S.B.: Epidemiological and Descriptive studies: Part II. Current clinical head injury research in the U.S. In Becker, D., and Povlishock, J.T. (Eds.): *Central Nervous System Trauma: Status Report* (pp. 45-53). Bethesda, National Institute of Health, National Institute of Neurological and Communicative Disorders and Stroke, 1985.

Matthews, D.J.: Pediatric head injuries. *Headlines News From the New Medico Head Injury System, May/June:* 8, 1987.

Meier, M.J., Benton, A.L., and Diller, L.: *Neuropsychological Rehabilitation.* New York, Guilford, 1987.

Mersky, H., and Woodforde, J.M.: Psychiatric sequelae of minor head injury. *Brain, 95:* 521, 1972.

Miller, E.: *Recovery and Management of Neuropsychological Impairments.* Chichester, Wiley, 1984.

National Head Injury Foundation: *An Educator's Manual.* Framingham, MA, Author, 1985.

Plum, F., and Posner, J.B.: *The Diagnosis of Stupor and Coma,* 3rd ed. Philadelphia, F.A. Davis, 1982.

Rimel, R., Giordini, B., Barth, J.T., Boll, T.J., and Jane, J.A.: Disability caused by minor head injury. *Neurosurgery,* 9: 221, 1981.

Rimel, R.W., and Jane, J.A. Characteristics of the Head-Injured Patient. In Rosenthal, M., Griffith, E., Bond, M., and Miller, J.: *Rehabilitation of the Head Injured Adult.* Philadelphia, F.A. Davis, 1983.

Rosenthal, M.: Traumatic Head Injury: Neurobehavioral Consequences. In Caplan, B. (Ed.): *Rehabilitation Psychology Desk Reference.* Rockville, MD, Aspen, 1987.

Savage, R., Cohen, S., Coyne, M., Fryer, J., and Harrington, D. (Speakers): *Educational Strategies: Secondary and Postsecondary Issues.* (Cassette Recording.) Framingham, MA, National Head Injury Foundation, 1985.

Sperry, R.W.: Lateral Specialization in the Surgically Separated Hemispheres. In Schmitt, F.O., and Worden, F.G. (Eds.): *The Neurosciences Third Study Program.* Cambridge, MIT Press, 1974.

Springer, S.P., and Deutsch, G.: *Left Brain Right Brain,* revised edition. New York, Freeman, 1985.

United States Department of Health and Human Services (Public Health Services), National Institute of Health: *Head Injury Hope Through Research.* Bethesda, Author, 1984.

Valenstein, E.S.: *Brain Control.* New York, Wiley, 1973.

Ylvisaker, M. (Ed.): *Head Injury Rehabilitation: Children and Adolescents.* San Diego, College-Hill, 1985.

INDEX